Jenny Tschiesche is a registered nutritionist, author of several family cookbooks and founder of LunchboxDoctor.com. Her lunchbox recipes have been shared thousands of times online and praised for the way they add variety to family diets and liven up lunchtimes.

JENNY TSCHIESCHE

Real
LUNCH
TIME
Food

A How To Book

ROBINSON

ROBINSON

First published in Great Britain in 2019
by Robinson

10 9 8 7 6 5 4 3 2 1

Copyright © Jenny Tschiesche, 2019

The moral right of the author has been
asserted.

A CIP catalogue record for this book
is available from the British Library.

ISBN: 978-1-47214-286-3

Typeset in Great Britain by
Mousemat Design Limited

Printed and bound in Great Britain by
Clays Ltd, Elcograf S.p.A.

Papers used by Robinson are from
well-managed forests and other
sustainable sources

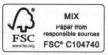

MIX
Paper from
responsible sources
FSC® C104740
www.fsc.org

Robinson
An imprint of
Little, Brown Book Group
Carmelite House
50 Victoria Embankment
London EC4Y 0DZ

An Hachette UK Company
www.hachette.co.uk

www.littlebrown.co.uk

The recommendations given in this
book are solely intended as education
and should not be taken as medical
advice.

y To Books are published by
inson, an imprint of Little,
wn Book Group. We welcome
oosals from authors who have
-hand experience of their
ects. Please set out the aims
ur book, its target market and
uggested contents in an email
owto@littlebrown.co.uk

Contents

Acknowledgements

I'd like to thank the following people for their support in creating this book. Thank you to my incredibly supportive family, friends and to my children's friends who willingly became new recipe guinea pigs. To my husband who I know is fed up of washing dishes and being asked for his opinion but rarely complains. To my eldest child who inspired me to start writing about and sharing recipes for healthy packed lunches in the first place. She still doesn't like sandwiches. To my youngest child who ensures I challenge myself and my explanations thanks to his constantly enquiring mind. To all the recipe testers involved in this book – Tina Foote, Rebecca Dandy, Malissa Berry, Anna Hemmings MBE, Ann and Andy Loder, Catherine Hamm, Mary Nash, Jo Keyes, Simone Gilbert, Megan Ormand. I'm extremely grateful to my literary agent Jane from Graham Maw Christie for believing in me and in the concept of this book. To my publisher Little, Brown Book Group for supporting me throughout the publishing process. Thank you one and all.

1 Introduction

Why You Should Read this Book

You may have picked up this book for several reasons. You may be one of the growing number of people taking their own lunches to school or work already, but you are running out of healthy ideas. You may be a parent who is keen to improve the nutritional balance of your child's packed lunches, but you either don't have the time or perhaps they don't share your enthusiasm for change. You may be teetering on the edge of making the decision to take your own lunches to work or school, but you're not really sure what to put in or even what equipment to buy to transport the food safely. Whichever of these best describes you, this book can help you take the next step. It is designed to explain the advantages of real lunchtime food, what constitutes a nutritionally balanced lunchtime meal and how best to transport this meal to work or school. Along the way you'll discover lots of top tips and ideas to help overcome hurdles and objections from those more particular about their lunchtime foods and brands.

For the past ten years I have been running lunchbox workshops all over the world, both as part of corporate wellbeing programmes and within schools. I am a UK-based nutritionist known as the Lunchbox Doctor. I shall bring to bear a wealth of knowledge on the subject of real food lunches and how to make lunch a healthier, more enjoyable and more nutritious meal.

What is Real Lunchtime Food?

Packed lunches provide you with an opportunity to eat foods that not only taste delicious but also provide nutritional and health benefits. Think food and not just fuel. Real food is minimally processed and maintains its natural integrity. Obvious examples include an apple, some milk or a boiled egg. Processed lunchtime foods such as crisps, cereal bars and pasties are the opposite of real lunchtime food.

While this book will certainly provide suggestions for shop-bought real foods, there are also numerous simple recipes. Where shop-bought real foods are concerned there's a simple rule of thumb – look for those with the fewest and most recognisable ingredients. An example would be lightly salted tortilla chips compared to a well-known brand of tangy cheese tortilla chips. The lightly salted tortillas contain more recognisable ingredients and fewer of them. These are a better option than the more processed tangy cheese flavour tortillas. See the ingredients labels below:

LIGHTLY SALTED
Whole Yellow Corn Kernels (75%), Sunflower Oil, Sea Salt (0.75%)

TANGY CHEESE
Corn (Maize), Vegetable Oils (Sunflower, Rapeseed, in varying proportions), Tangy Cheese Flavour [Flavourings (from Milk), Wheat Powder (from Milk), Wheat Flour (contains Calcium, Iron, Niacin, Thiamin), Salt, Cheese Powder (from Milk), Buttermilk Powder, Potassium Chloride, Flavour Enhancer (Monosodium Glutamate), Milk Protein, Dextrose, Acids (Lactic Acid, Citric Acid), Colours (Paprika Extract, Annatto, Plain Caramel), Spice, Sugar, Skimmed Milk Powder]

As far as recipes are concerned, here's a flavour of what to expect: crustless quiches, beetroot hummus, pea and mint soup, raspberry chia flapjacks and tuna tacos. There are real food and drink recipes galore, but allow me to reassure you that the focus is on maximum output for minimal input. Few of us have the time nor the inclination to spend hours creating a culinary masterpiece for our own lunch and certainly not our children's lunches too.

Why Should We Eat Real Foods?

We 'eat with our eyes', which to my mind means foods that look colourful and tasty in the lunchbox are far more likely to be consumed and enjoyed. But the most colourful part of the lunchbox-suitable foods on offer in supermarkets is often the packaging, and not the food itself. At the heart of this book is the guiding principle that we have an innate desire as human beings to want to eat foods that look more visually appealing. A study in the late 1970s showed that when we find food more visually appealing, not only do we enjoy it more, we also absorb more nutrients from it.

Multiple studies show improvements in afternoon performance and in schoolchildren's test scores when we have consumed a nutritionally balanced lunch. This is such an important association to make. The right food choices can make a difference to how well we can do our jobs or how efficiently our children can concentrate and study in the afternoons. In short: making better food choices makes for a better, more productive us.

What's Wrong with 'Unreal' Foods?

Supermarkets offer meal deals designed for convenience and value – they are often the cheapest way to buy the largest quantity of food. Yet, the options available tend to be limited to a sandwich, a sugary snack and a drink. At the same time the number of bakery retailers and fast food franchises offering their own lunchtime meal deals is on the rise. These seem to limit the range of foods on offer predominantly to sandwiches, pasties and pasta salads. Meanwhile, the most common children's lunchbox foods are ham or cheese sandwiches on white bread, a packet of crisps and a cake or biscuit, with the odd piece of fruit which often comes home uneaten.

Pick any one of these combinations – the white-bread cheese or ham sandwich, crisps and chocolate biscuit combination or the chicken mayonnaise baguette and fruit juice combination, for example – and you'll find a meal distinctly lacking in vegetables, quality proteins and complex (slow-releasing) carbohydrates. What these meals will provide is an instant energy hit followed by an energy low as the refined carbohydrates turn into sugar (glucose) in the body, and the body responds in kind, bringing energy levels down with it. Furthermore, these meals are unable to contribute health-giving nutrients due to being predominantly processed foods, designed for enjoyment at the time of eating but not for long-term energy nor health.

Where school or work canteens are concerned, the range of foods on offer is often not optimally balanced because their focus is on providing the food they believe most people will eat – they are a business in their own right, so they don't want waste. If the majority of people will eat what's on offer, even if it's not ideal nutritionally, then the caterers don't end up throwing food away. For this reason, many schools have removed or no longer fill the salad bar, and pizzas and paninis are increasingly on offer throughout the lunchtime period, if not beyond.

Packed Lunches are Here to Stay

Increasing numbers of adults are taking packed lunches to work and we're talking about our lunch more than ever. The hashtags #lunch and #lunchbox receive tens of millions of hits on Instagram year after year and are growing in popularity. Adults are increasingly moving away from the traditional sandwich, crisps and fruit combination, opening a world of nutritional possibilities. It's not uncommon to take leftovers from the previous evening's meal in an insulated flask to work. That's certainly something to be encouraged from a nutritional and effort perspective. Increasingly, adults are also looking for influences from other food cultures, such as the use of Japanese bento boxes and Indian tiffin boxes, as well as taste influences from Asia, the Middle East and the Mediterranean. These influences are slowly finding their way into children's lunchboxes too.

While the number of children taking lunches to school is fairly stable, the focus on a healthier lunch for children is certainly increasing. As parents become more aware of the negative impact on energy levels, satiety and even immunity of poorer food choices, such as crisps and chocolate, so there is a greater focus on adding vegetables to lunches and reducing sugary snacks. There has also been a rise in the number of social media groups that have sprung up to provide ideas and support. In some schools a packed lunch is the only option, as there is no canteen and so the focus must be on that meal being a nutritionally balanced one.

Packed Lunches are a Global Phenomenon

Although they go by different names in different countries they're based on the same concepts. They are cost effective, easily packed and transported to work or school. In the US, they're known as 'bag lunches', Matpakke in Norway and certain regions even have their own name for a packed lunch, such as the 'pack up' in Yorkshire in the UK. In India, couriers known as 'dabbawallas' take the tiffin (lunchboxes) to workers all over the city of Mumbai from their homes in time for lunch. In Japan, a bento box is used to present the fresh foods in a visually appealing and easily accessible way for workers and school children alike. These lunches are designed to make people's lives simpler and to ensure that lunchtime is not a wasted meal opportunity. That's exactly what this book aims to do for you. To show you how easily portable lunches (whatever name you want to give them) can be created and transported to work so that they're still nutritious, enticing and delicious come lunchtime.

Packed lunches have come a long way since their humble beginnings. Once the only option for blue-collar workers like miners and builders during the late 1800s for cost reasons, the packed lunch has been through a roller-coaster ride through the years. Not only has it waxed and waned in terms of its popularity, but the sorts of foods you'd find in a lunch have almost come full circle. Now people are getting back to the foods once taken to work in the mines or building sites by those blue-collar workers, foods like hard-boiled eggs, raw egetables, meat, pies and sourdough bread (because that is all that would have existed then). Added to that is a new trend looking towards other food cultures and adopting their 'best practices' as our own is appearing. Rice paper wraps in place of dough-based wraps, adding probiotic-rich kefir to a 'milkshake' or serving root vegetable-based hummus might not have been common back in the early days of lunchboxes but these are the sorts of ideas you are going to find here. This book is about time-saving, delicious, real-food lunchbox ideas that are nutritionally balanced.

Think Food Not Fuel

If we think of food not as fuel but as nourishment, we start to think of the lunchbox in a different context. We are not just looking for foods to provide the calories we need or the energy we require but also the nutrients – vitamins, minerals, antioxidants – that can nourish the body. For example, calcium helps build bones, regulates blood pressure, keeps cells communicating and keeps muscles working optimally. Magnesium plays an important role in energy production, blood sugar control and muscle and nerve function. Anthocyanins in red and purple foods have neuroprotective effects and improve vision. None of these nutrients provide fuel. They do nourish the body though. We don't want to miss out on the opportunity that lunchtime provides to nourish, not just refuel.

The information in this book should not be overwhelming. The contents are designed simply to explain why anyone might want to make changes to their packed lunches or those of their children. There are sections that will address any questions or concerns you may have. There are chapters outlining what to look for in terms of healthier products in shops and supermarkets. There's information on how best to transport your lunch to work or school, from a practical and environmental standpoint. There are recipes galore, but they are not overcomplicated. They have been designed to fit into our already busy lives, with simple, clear steps and few ingredients.

Over the past ten years, since my eldest child first went to school and I went out to work as a nutritionist running events and workshops all over the country, we've made countless lunchboxes as a family. After setting up Lunchbox Doctor, a business specialising in nutrition education, I feel like I have answered every conceivable question and objection regarding the subject of healthy lunchboxes. This book truly reflects that depth and breadth of experience.

If you are looking for lunchbox inspiration and want to focus on taste and health when it comes to lunchtime choices, but don't have much time on your hands, then keep reading. This is the book for you.

2 Lunchbox Planning

Lunchbox Planning Made Easy

Planning a balanced lunchtime meal doesn't need to be difficult. However, the task is made harder by the number of foods marketed as 'ideal for lunchboxes' available in supermarkets and take-away food outlets, many of which are made up of refined carbohydrates, of low or poor protein value and lacking in nutrient density. It's the misleading information and alluring messaging that surrounds us that makes balanced lunches harder to achieve. Yet, if we have learned one thing about nutrition from mainstream media in recent years, it is that refined carbohydrates leave us feeling low in energy just hours after we have eaten them and often lead us to crave more of the same.

We need to be careful not to load our packed lunches with crisps, breads, cakes, biscuits, and, of course, we need to avoid too many added sugars. It's also important to make sure we have enough protein, calcium, some vegetables, fruit and a drink too. There's a mental checklist to go through so that you ensure your lunch is nutritionally balanced. Our lives are sufficiently busy already though, so if you find using a mental checklist adds to the load, then using a physical lunchbox-planning template can really help.

Lunchbox Bingo – a New Lunchbox Planning Framework

Lunchbox Bingo is a really simple planning template to help you make nutritionally balanced packed lunches. You might not use it for ever but it's a great way of getting into the habit of planning a well-rounded, healthy meal on a daily basis. Lunchbox Bingo is also a great way of reinvigorating things whenever you find your lunches are becoming samey or when you find yourself falling back into familiar habits of sandwich plus accompaniments. An additional benefit to using this planning template is that you tend not to waste food because each day you know what is going into each lunchbox and you can buy the right amounts of the right kinds of food accordingly.

Lunchbox Bingo is as useful a planning tool for children as it is for adults. In fact, I initially developed it because I wanted to find a way of getting my own children both involved in and empowered by the decision-making process when it came to packing their lunches.

After some time and through trial and error this worksheet proved to be our lunchbox planning saviour. It's a great way to give them a say in what they eat. They could choose their own lunches provided they wrote down what they wanted – in the early days I helped them with the writing part – and so long as each of the food groups had at least one tick in it for each day of the week. We still use this system today and I recommend it to adults and children alike. It can be used in physical form to write up lunchbox menu plans a week at a time but when you're used to the format you might choose to use it simply as a checklist when shopping or making lunches.

The Six Components of a Balanced Lunchbox

For those new to the process the six components of a balanced lunchbox fall into the following categories, each providing a predominant health benefit:

1. CARBOHYDRATE – energy foods
2. PROTEIN – repair and growth foods
3. CALCIUM – for strong teeth and bones
4. FRUIT – to boost immunity
5. VEGETABLE – to boost immunity
6. DRINK – to improve concentration

How to Use Lunchbox Bingo

This process should inspire you to think of foods you'd like to eat each day of the week, while also ticking off the food groups that each food belongs to. For example, a Tuna Pasta Salad would tick off the following boxes: carbohydrate, protein, and if there were vegetables in there then the vegetable box too:

	Carbohydrate	Protein	Calcium	Fruit	Vegetable	Drink
DAY						
Tuna pasta salad	✓	✓			✓	

Ensure that on each day of the week there is at least one tick in each column so each of the food groups is covered. That equates to a full house in lunchbox bingo!

A whole lunchtime meal might look like this:

	Carbohydrate	Protein	Calcium	Fruit	Vegetable	Drink
DAY						
Tuna pasta salad	✓	✓			✓	
Hummus and carrot sticks		✓	✓		✓	
Apple with yogurt and honey	✓	✓	✓	✓		
Water						✓

In order to effectively plan real lunchtime meals using the Lunchbox Bingo template (see p.12), it helps if you can develop an understanding of which foods fall primarily into which food group. For example, chicken is a protein and carrots are vegetables, while hummus is both a protein and provides calcium. A fruit and vegetable smoothie would be fruit, vegetable and a drink.

Which Food for Which Group?

In order to select those foods you enjoy most from each food group, use the following as a prompt:

Lunchbox Carbohydrates

Filled pitta pockets

Baked pitta chips

Traditional flatbreads – always read the ingredients label. Those with fewer and more recognisable ingredients are preferable to those with an extensive list of less recognisable ingredients

Sourdough or rye bread

Wholegrain or gluten-free pasta with a choice of sauce

New potatoes in their skins, as mini jacket potatoes with fillings or in a potato salad

Flapjacks

Crackers, oatcakes, rye crackers, buckwheat crackers

Popcorn – home-made or shop-bought

Lightly salted tortilla chips

Root vegetable crisps/chips – home-made or shop-bought

Roasted root vegetables

Root vegetable soups

Lunchbox Proteins

Cold, lean roasted meats, such as beef, pork, lamb or chicken

Chorizo, ham, bacon, sausages, bresaola, Parma ham

Dips made from pulses, for example hummus or white bean dip
Cheese, cream cheese, cottage cheese, quark, yogurt, kefir
Good-quality sausages – ideally 90 per cent meat or more
Eggs – boiled, or made into an omelette, frittata or savoury slices
Seeds or nuts
Pulses – lentils, chickpeas, beans and peas
Tofu or tempeh

Lunchbox Calcium Sources
Carton of milk
Yogurt or kefir, as a dessert or as part of a dip
Cheese, cottage cheese, quark
Dark green lettuce leaves
Kale chips
Spinach, as part of a cooked dish
Broccoli spears
Sesame seed bars
Seed bars
Hummus
Nut bars
Flapjacks with seeds and nuts

Note: Always check that nuts are allowed in your child's school.

Lunchbox Vegetables
Crudités, for example carrots, peppers, cucumber sticks, sugar snap peas,
    baby sweetcorn
Vegetable muffins and flapjacks
Olives
Root vegetables, either as juices or grated in salads or baked goods
Sweetcorn – on the cob or kernels mixed into salads or sandwich fillings
Salad leaves combined with other salad vegetables
Vegetable dips
Vegetable-based pasta sauces
Cooked meals in a flask, for example soups, casseroles, stews, curries.
    These can be leftovers from the previous evening's meal
Root vegetable crisps
Savoury vegetable pancakes and slices

Lunchbox Fruits

Banana, apple, orange, pear, grapefruit
Berries, cherries
Nectarines, peaches
Figs
Dried fruit
Fruit muffins and flapjacks
Fruit purées
Smoothies
Fruity shakes
Fruit salad
Fruity chia puddings
Fruit crumbles

Lunchbox Drinks

Carton of milk
Fruit smoothies or milkshakes – home-made or shop-bought
Fruit and vegetable smoothies – home-made or shop-bought
Vegetable smoothies – home-made or shop-bought
Fruit juice and water mixed together
Water

Lunchbox Bingo Chart

All you need to do is create your own copy of this template ahead of the next week of lunches and fill it in. This planning sheet will help you organise your food shopping list for the week, and will mean you have less food waste.

Lunchtime Bingo

	Carbohydrate	Protein	Calcium	Fruit	Vegetable	Drink
MONDAY						
TUESDAY						
WEDNESDAY						
THURSDAY						
FRIDAY						

Key: ✓ Nutritional Component Included

Sample Menu Plan #1
Lunchtime Bingo

	Carbohydrate	Protein	Calcium	Fruit	Vegetable	Drink
MONDAY						
Moroccan lamb plus natural yogurt		✓	✓		✓	
Flatbread	✓					
Lighter Eton mess	✓	✓	✓	✓		
Cucumber water						✓
TUESDAY						
Chicken curry		✓			✓	
Courgette chips					✓	
Spicy bircher	✓	✓	✓	✓		
Water						✓
WEDNESDAY						
Courgette and sun-dried tomato bread	✓	✓	✓	✓	✓	
Roasted salted beetroot					✓	
Berry coulis and yogurt		✓	✓	✓		
Strawberry banana milkshake			✓	✓		✓
THURSDAY						
Crustless quiche Lorraine		✓	✓			
Beetroot hummus and oatcakes	✓	✓	✓		✓	
Spicy roasted chickpeas		✓				
Protein yogurt with protein pancake	✓	✓	✓	✓		
Water						✓
FRIDAY						
Rocket pesto on pasta	✓		✓		✓	
Sweetcorn and paprika fritters	✓	✓			✓	
Fruity kefir shake		✓	✓	✓		✓

Key: ✓ Nutritional Component Included

Sample Menu Plan #2
Lunchtime Bingo

	Carbohydrate	Protein	Calcium	Fruit	Vegetable	Drink
MONDAY						
Mexican tuna with nachos	✓	✓			✓	
Berry chia pudding		✓	✓	✓		
Batons of carrot and pepper					✓	
Carrot and mango smoothie				✓	✓	✓
TUESDAY						
Chocolate bean chilli soup		✓			✓	
Kale chips			✓		✓	
Chocolate orange flapjack	✓					
Watermelon froth				✓		✓
WEDNESDAY						
Lentil bolognese on pasta	✓	✓			✓	
Sweet and spicy seed mix		✓	✓			
Green smoothie				✓	✓	✓
THURSDAY						
Beef and vegetable burgers		✓			✓	
Halloumi baked fries		✓	✓			
Popcorn	✓					
Yogurt with apple and orange compote		✓	✓	✓		
Water						✓
FRIDAY						
Savoury oat slice	✓	✓	✓		✓	
Red pepper hummus and celery batons		✓	✓		✓	
Blueberry and banana smoothie				✓		✓

Key: ✓ Nutritional Component Included

Lunchbox Making Basics

Going Shopping

Hands up if you find shopping for food a drag? For many it is their least favourite chore. The last thing you want is to be traipsing round the supermarket looking for obscure, expensive ingredients that even the shop assistants didn't know they sold. The majority of ingredients listed in this book are widely available in most supermarkets. Where I offer ideas for alternatives I do so with good reason: generally to help those with intolerances or allergies to certain ingredients.

Where lunchbox foods are concerned, I urge you to read the ingredients labels. The rule of thumb is that fewer ingredients mean that the food has more nutritional value. We have all been there, holding two seemingly identical items in the supermarket: one with health claims and benefits plastered all over the packaging, but it contains twenty-three ingredients; while the other is wrapped in plain packaging, is cheaper and has just four ingredients. Which is healthier, we wonder? Is it the one telling us it is through its marketing messaging or is it the understated product? Check the ingredients labels and remember that less is more.

When purchasing lunchbox foods, I'd recommend:

1   Choosing ingredients or foods that are, where possible, unprocessed. These tend to fall into just a handful of categories: pulses, beans and peas; meat, fish and poultry; vegetables, fruit, dairy (milk, cheese, plain yogurt, butter); and wholegrains, nuts and seeds.
2   Avoiding food items that claim they are ideal for lunchboxes. They rarely are. What the manufacturers often mean by this is that the food is individually wrapped and contains preservatives to give it a longer life.
3   Steering clear of any product that has sugar as its main ingredient.
4   Looking above and below eye level in supermarkets. Bigger brands and processed foods will pay more to be at optimal level for customers to see. You may need to look above and below this level to find the better, healthier products. Remember, eye level is different for adults and children, so look above and below eye

level for the items you're seeking, i.e. for your own or your child's lunchbox.

5   Finding your local farm shop, butcher, delicatessen, greengrocer or bakery as you may find they have better offers, better quality produce and more seasonal produce. Increasingly, they are also offering delivery schemes that make your busy life so much easier.

Ingredients

Being able to produce healthy, nutritionally balanced lunches with minimal fuss requires the right ingredients to be in the house in the first place. Here are some essentials, many of which will appear in my lunchbox recipes:

STORE CUPBOARD

Pulses, peas and lentils, chickpeas, white beans

Seeds: pumpkin, sunflower, pine nuts, chia, ground flaxseed

Nuts: almonds – whole or ground, walnuts, cashews

Popcorn kernels

Flours: spelt, coconut, buckwheat, gluten-free, gram (chick pea) flour or pea flour

Tins: chopped tomatoes/passata, soup, fish, pulses, dahl, coconut milk, coconut cream, fruit in fruit juice

Pesto: red or green

Oats

Quinoa

Pasta: gnocchi, gluten-free, wholegrain spelt, chickpea, lentil

Rice paper wraps and/or nori (seaweed) sheets

Nut butters: peanut, almond

Sweet things: Raw honey, maple syrup, stevia, coconut sugar, yacon syrup (optional)

Oils: coconut, avocado, extra virgin olive

FRIDGE

Greek yogurt, kefir, drinking yogurt

Butter

Milk: dairy and non-dairy

Cream: dairy and non-dairy

Green vegetables: lettuce, broccoli, avocado, courgette, cucumber, kale, rocket, spinach, lettuce

Colourful vegetables: carrot, sweet potato, butternut squash, pepper, beetroot

Other vegetables: mushroom, garlic, onion (red and brown)

Fruit: tomato, apple, berry, nectarine, peach, pear, banana

Citrus fruit: lemon, lime, orange

Cheeses: feta, halloumi, Cheddar, pecorino, mozzarella, quark, Emmental, Gruyére, cottage cheese

Meat and fish: Chorizo, ham, bacon, sausages, bresaola, smoked fish – ideally those without nitrates

Fresh herbs

Flavours: apple cider vinegar, sun-dried
    tomatoes, tomato paste, mustard,
    spices, herbs, stock cubes, soy
    sauce/tamari (gluten-free soy
    sauce), bouillon, curry paste, miso,
    chipotle paste
Rice noodles
Olives
Cacao or cocoa powder
Baking: bicarbonate of soda, baking
    powder
Arrowroot powder
Vanilla extract
Eggs
Seasoning: sea salt, pepper
Crackers: oat, rye

FREEZER
Berries
Bananas: peeled and sliced
Mango
Spinach
Garlic
Ginger
Herbs
Peas
Sweetcorn

Equipment
It pays to have the right equipment for preparing varied and
nutritious lunches. The following items are recommended for a well-
equipped lunchbox-making kitchen.

- Food processor
- Roasting trays of various sizes
- Large, medium and small saucepans
- Frying pan
- Bread tins
- Brownie tin with 12 holes/sections
- Muffin tin
- Quality knives
- Grater
- Peeler and julienne peeler

5 Ways to Stress-free Packed Lunches
One of the most common reasons for lunchbox packing to be a
stressful activity is a lack of advanced planning. Like most things in
life, a little planning goes a long way. To this end I have focused all the
planning and preparation you need for smart, efficient and stress-
free lunch packing, into five top tips.

1 Plan lunchboxes before you go food shopping

Writing out a plan for lunches is highly recommended. You can find the Lunchbox Bingo planning template on p.12. It is designed to make the task of lunchbox planning more enjoyable, interactive and to take the stress out of packing lunches. Once you've created the plan, simply add the items to your food shopping list so you know you'll have the right foods and ingredients in the house to make healthy, nutritionally balanced lunches.

2 Prepare food in advance

On a weekend or during the week, if you have some time:

- Make a big batch or two of pasta sauce. Both tomato-based sauces and green pesto are easy to make and freeze well. You can even freeze the sauce in portions so you only need to defrost enough for that day each time.
- Batch cook hot meals or soups as and when you have some time. Freeze in portion sizes. These can easily be defrosted overnight and heated up the following morning then transported to work or school in a flask.
- Make a batch of flapjacks, slices, muffins, biscuits or cakes for lunches throughout the week. Store in an airtight container so they last.
- Make some pancakes, savoury slices, crunchy snacks.
- Prepare a fruit purée or coulis to add to yogurts or some alternative puddings to yogurt ahead of time. It's so much easier to grab one of these pre-prepared puddings and go rather than have to make it up each morning.
- Wash and chop some vegetables and fruit for the next few days. You could wash some cherry tomatoes, chop mango into cubes, peel and chop carrots into sticks, cube some melon. If you are worried about these going dry, either cover them in a damp tea towel or store them in the fridge in sealed containers.

3 Make double

Whenever you are making a meal, cook more than you are going to eat then serve up the leftovers in lunchboxes the next day, either hot in a Thermos flask or cold.

Some ideas for hot leftovers include shepherd's pie, cottage pie, fish pie, curry, stew, casserole, tagine, roast dinner, soup or spaghetti bolognese.

Some ideas for cold leftovers: roast meats, salads, home-made pizza, pasta and sauce, curry.

4 Freeze for later

Freezing foods for when you really need them is a great way to make sure you don't fall into the trap of having to pay for a lunch simply because you don't have anything at home to pack.

- It's helpful to always have sliced bread and pitta bread in the freezer to defrost on a morning when you suddenly realise you've run out.
- Hummus can be frozen too, but the key to ensuring it stays moist is to cover the hummus in a layer of olive oil before freezing.
- Cheese can be frozen in portions. This does change its texture a little but in an emergency it's useful to have.
- Cold cooked meats, such as ham, turkey, chicken and chorizo, can be frozen if wrapped tightly in airtight packaging, and if using it in baked goods the texture change won't matter anyway.
- Freeze home-made muffins or indeed the dough for biscuits. The muffins can simply be defrosted on the morning you need them. Biscuit dough can be halved and some frozen when making a batch of biscuits then defrosted and baked fresh for lunches.
- Full-fat Greek yogurt can be frozen too. Those with lower fat and greater water content do not freeze well, however.
- Having frozen berries, frozen peeled banana slices, frozen mango and frozen avocado can make a quick smoothie a possibility.

5 Saviour foods

It's a good idea to keep some longer-life foods in the house just in case. Some ideas are included in the table overleaf.

Carbohydrate	Protein	Calcium	Fruit	Vegetable	Drink
Wholegrain crackers in sealed packages	Cartons or tins of beans	Nuts	Cartons or tins of soup	Tinned fruit	Long life milk (dairy and non-dairy, e.g.
	Tinned fish	Seeds	Tinned sweetcorn	Dried fruit	almond,
Small bags of popcorn	Ready cooked quinoa	Tahini	Jars of antipasti, e.g.	Foil packs or jars of olives	oat, rice)
Corn chips		Nut and seed butters	sun-dried tomatooo,		Fruit juice
		Sachets of Miso soup	and roasted peppers		Fizzy water

Some emergency lunchbox food ideas:
- When you get caught out because you have very little in the house there's always soup – blend some vegetables and add some stock with meat or pulses.
- Or if you have leftover cooked vegetables and some fresh eggs then individually baked frittatas (see p.43) make great lunchbox food.
- A trail mix can be made from nuts, seeds and dried fruit.
- A simple drink can be created from fruit juice and fizzy water.

3 Transporting Lunch to Work or School

The Importance of How You Pack

We could all throw lunch into a bag and take it to work or school but would it be truly appealing to the eye and the appetite come lunchtime? Workplaces sometimes have fridges, but schools rarely do. Keeping a lunch looking, smelling and tasting great is important because a few black bananas, leaked yogurts and squashed tomatoes later, you'll be ready to throw in the towel as far as packing lunches is concerned. It's not just the look, smell and taste of the lunch though. It's important also to consider the temperature of the food – transporting your lunch in an insulated container is imperative.

Thinking about the Environment

You may want to think about how the equipment you use to transport your lunch impacts on the environment. Many of us are trying to make greener choices. If we want to address this issue, we can use fewer non-recyclable packaging options, such as plastics, foil, cling film, and instead buy reusable and recyclable packaging. For some people, reducing their environmental impact and reducing the amount of non-recyclable waste they contribute to the environment will be their main reason and purpose for making packed lunches in the first place.

Cost Considerations

As with most things in life there will be cost considerations too. You may be the kind of person who wants the latest and greatest lunchbox equipment, but there are some less costly and perfectly suitable lunchboxes, tins, bento boxes, insulated bottles that are totally fit for purpose. While you don't necessarily want to be investing loads of money, you don't want to scrimp on quality. Lunchboxes tend to get a great deal of use, so if you are intending to use your equipment multiple times a week or even every day, it's going to get bashed about a bit. Consider also that when you wash the equipment each day, its seals and surfaces will start to degrade over time.

The most important considerations when purchasing lunchbox equipment are:

- Freshness
- Temperature
- Appearance
- Cost
- Environmental impact

Why not consider the following items:

Insulated Lunch Bag/Box
You want the lunch that you pack to taste as good at lunchtime as you imagined it would when you packed it. An insulated lunch bag or box will go a long way to keeping the lunch at the right temperature, at the same time as providing protection to the food itself.

If you are interested in reducing the environmental impact of your lunch bag or box, look for those made with eco-friendly materials and lined with BPA-free plastic. The materials should be made obvious at the point of purchase.

Cold Packs
Cold packs are fairly standard wherever you buy them. The thickness does play a part in how long the food within the lunchbox is kept cool though. There is a trade-off between the thickness of the pack and the amount of food you need to keep cool and for how long. For this reason, it is worth having a range of slimmer and wider packs for different occasions and seasons.

Flasks
An insulated flask is an incredibly worthwhile investment. The benefits of having one are that you can:

- Use up leftovers from meals cooked the previous evening
- Batch cook meals at weekends and apportion one flaskful per day, freezing some portions for the latter part of the week
- In an emergency, heat up and serve tinned or long-life food, such as soup, low-sugar baked beans, lentil dahl, chickpea curry, bean chilli
- Keep baked foods, such as quiche, frittatas and muffins, warm until lunch
- Transport home-made soups, stews, chillies, pasta dishes to school or work

Simply being able to take cooked food that requires no specific storage at school or work and no reheating means you open up a whole range of options for packed lunches. Transporting cooked meals also means you are likely to save money because the overheads and profit of the canteen or shop are factored into the cost of any meal you purchase away from home. That is simply not the case with a home-cooked meal. See The Value of Insulated Flasks (p.96) for more on the benefits of using flasks, and how to use them effectively, and how to look after them.

Insulated Water Bottle

The world of water bottles has progressed considerably in recent years. There are now a range of good-quality but reasonably priced insulated water bottles on the market. They are created with double-wall insulation with an airless vacuum in between. That means they can keep hot liquids hot and cold liquids cold.

What's more, from a health perspective, drinking from a stainless-steel bottle – as opposed to a plastic one that has often been sat out in the sun – means that the liquid inside tastes better. That's because plastic often retains the smell of the drinks that we put in them. They also retain the smell of the soaps and detergents that are used to clean them. While there are aluminium bottles on the market, aluminium reacts with the liquid in the bottle and this can be responsible for the metallic taste that often results. Even if the aluminium bottle claims to have a lining, they often corrode or flake, leaving us susceptible to harm.

Insulated bottles are free of a chemical called BPA that has been established as a hormone disruptor[1]. It is recommended that you purchase bottles that are made from stainless steel, which is an alloy of chromium and iron, and does not release any chemicals or react with drinks to create funny metallic concoctions.

Insulated water bottles are not limited to transporting cold drinks to school or work. They can also transport hot drinks. A list of possibilities include both cold and hot options:

- Tea
- Coffee
- Herbal tea

[1] Rubins, BS. (2011) https://www.ncbi.nlm.nih.gov/pubmed/21605673

- Mint leaves in water
- Sliced cucumber, citrus fruits in water
- Ice-cold water
- Watered-down juice
- A selection of home-made drinks and smoothies – check out the chapter DRINKS FOR CONCENTRATION (p.194)

Reusable Food Pouches

These food pouches are ideal for those wanting to serve yogurt, smoothies or purées (vegetable, fruit or both combined) in the lunchbox but not wanting the expense nor the environmental cost of buying the single-use versions with food already packed in them from supermarkets.

These reusable pouches are easy to fill, clean, and the food within is secure as they have a wide zip-lock opening/closing. They are freezer-safe, allowing for the contents to be frozen and the pouch to be used as the cold pack in the lunch. The contents of the pouch can then gently defrost in time for lunch.

You should seek out brands that are BPA-, PVC-, lead- and phthalate-free. Ideally, they'd also be recyclable.

Bento Boxes

A bento box is a lunchbox that contains a variety of different foods, presented in different compartments. The bento box originates in Japan and its name is derived from a Japanese word meaning 'convenience'. You can pack whatever you like into a bento box though; it doesn't have to be Japanese food.

The advantages of a bento box are that you can see exactly what you have to eat. There's nothing missing or hidden. What you see is what you get. Rather like a buffet of colourful food you might see on holiday, it's a very appealing way for food to be presented. Given that all the food is on show and it looks visually appealing, it is more likely that everything will get eaten in one sitting.

Conversely, it is easier to see when the lunch is not colourful and visually appealing enough – remember, we eat with our eyes – or if it is missing a particular food group.

There are a wide variety of bento boxes designed for adults on the market with larger compartments marked by dividers. They are available in both stainless steel and durable, safe plastics.

For children there are an even wider variety of bento-style boxes on the market. Some have labels and diagrams to suggest which food group should go in which compartment of the box and how much should be packed for the child. These are very useful, especially if you are new to packing lunches with your child. Some of these bento-style boxes directly reflect the categories in the Lunchbox Bingo template used for planning lunchboxes – for more information look at the LUNCHBOX PLANNING (p.7) section of this book.

Lunch Pots and Tins

We have already covered the advantages of stainless steel over plastic, but there are a range of lunchbox pots on the market to suit all budgets, and reusing a plastic container over and over is far better for the environment than using disposable packaging each time. That said, stainless steel pots are extremely durable, 100 per cent recyclable and with fewer opportunities for bacteria to accumulate and less risk of contamination.

Small, medium and large pots can be useful for a variety of lunchbox items and provide a layer of protection when transporting fragile food items such as home-made biscuits, cakes, quiche and salads. Where some bento boxes (but certainly not all) may leak in between compartments, individually packed foods in separate pots won't. Ripe mango, soft cheese and moist cucumber don't taste so good when all their juices have merged.

When selecting lunchbox pots or tins for transporting food to work or school, be sure to check the lids. They must be secure enough that nothing leaks out but not so secure that they are difficult to open.

Reusable Fabric Wraps – Sandwiches

British children alone throw away 800 million bits of foil or cling film per year. So how can we ensure we throw away less packaging? Reusable fabric sandwich wraps can help. They come in a variety of designs, shapes, sizes and ways of opening and closing. The best are those that are made ethically and to a high standard with fabric outer layers and safe, plastic inner layers – making the product easy to wipe clean.

Reusable Fabric Bags – Snacks

Small fabric snack bags are also available. They make their own contribution to reducing plastics as they render individually packed crisps/chips unnecessary. You can buy larger bags of snacks and apportion a suitable handful into the snack bag as the lunch is being prepped. These bags are also useful for more sturdy biscuits and cakes.

Beeswax Wrappers
These are a reusable, biodegradable wrap for lunchbox foods. They are easy to clean, with a little soap and cold water, and are naturally adhesive and so wrap around the food tightly preventing air from getting in and spoiling your lunch. There are quite a few online companies selling these now as well as some artisan stores. Once you have used your wrap you can also simply throw it onto the compost heap.

Paper Food Bags
If you want to use less cling film and foil but cannot get on with wraps for sandwiches and snacks, then recyclable paper bags are an option. These bags are ideal for transporting snacks, biscuits, muffins, nuts, crisps/chips, sandwiches and much more. There are a few brands of paper sandwich bag on the market now. They should be made from 100 per cent FSC Certified, unbleached paper, be biodegradable and landfill safe. Be careful as some bags on the market are treated with petroleum-based paraffin wax or use toxic glues to bind them.

4 Not Just Sandwiches

Out with White Sliced Bread
The sales of sliced bread are falling. Over the past five years, sales of bread in the UK have declined 12 per cent[2]. The reason for this is a trend towards adults generally wanting to eat foods lower in refined carbohydrates and increasing concerns about the health effects of too much gluten. Consumers also want more choice. As workers compete for the best lunch in the office, sandwiches feature less and less and in their place are salads, protein bowls, frittatas and leftovers from the night before.

Moving on from Sandwiches for Children
Where children are concerned it's a different story. The sliced bread sandwich is still a key feature. In fact, 88 per cent of children's lunchboxes contain a sandwich[3]. Most lunchbox sandwiches, 87 per cent according to one study[4], are on sliced white bread.

The most common sandwich filling is ham. Yet, it will come as no surprise to find that a ham sandwich on white bread is not the most nutritious lunch. It contains just 1g of dietary fibre, as well as 35 per cent of an adult's recommended daily intake of sodium and 70 per cent of that recommended for a 4–6-year-old. Of course, there's an opportunity with a sandwich to include some vegetables, perhaps some lettuce, tomato or cucumber. Though it seems few children like this option as much as just plain ham!

While packed lunches without a sandwich might seem a bit strange to begin with, replacing the sandwich with an alternative can provide an opportunity to broaden the nutritional profile of the lunchbox and break the cycle of daily sandwiches. You will find some alternatives to sandwich options in this chapter.

Why Sliced White Bread Causes Energy Lows
The reason there has been a decline in sales of sliced white bread is

[2] https://www.theguardian.com/business/2017/nov/11/are-uks-leading-bakers-toast-bread-sales-fall-costs-rise

[3] http://www.leedsbeckett.ac.uk/news/1014-survey-reveals-parents-choices-in-providing-childrens-packed-lunches/

[4] http://news.bbc.co.uk/1/hi/health/3192079.stm

that we now understand more about how it can contribute to a short-term energy surge followed by an energy low. Just look at this diagram and you'll see how quickly this reaction occurs.

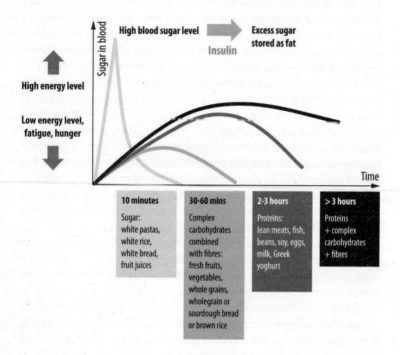

It goes without saying that energy surges followed by abrupt energy lows are not a good thing, whether you're a child or an adult. Low energy in the middle of the afternoon means a lack of productivity and concentration. Ask team leaders holding team meetings mid-afternoon or a teacher trying to help six-year-olds master subtraction in an afternoon lesson, and you'll hear a familiar tale.

Chorleywood Bread Process

That's not to say a sandwich cannot still be a part of a balanced lunchbox. It's just important to choose a type of bread that's not going to result in energy lows. The vast majority of bread eaten – as much as 76 per cent – as part of a packed lunch is made using the

Chorleywood bread-making method[5]. This method came about in 1961 as a way of producing a large number of loaves, quickly, cheaply and from British wheat, which is low in protein due to the nature of the British climate. This process reduced the time required to make bread as well as the labour input. It involves milling the wheat in high-speed steel mills at high temperatures, a process that breaks apart the starches making it easier for the enzymes and improvers to work on the flour but in so doing reducing the nutritional value.

Bread made using this process has a far more dramatic effect on blood-sugar levels than more traditionally made loaves. This can be measured in terms of glycaemic index, which is a figure given to carbohydrate foods indicating the ability of that food to raise the levels of sugar in the blood. Chorleywood bread has a far higher glycaemic index than traditionally made loaves. Furthermore, these loaves are created in such a way that the gluten in the wheat is released very quickly to produce a stiff dough. This bombards our digestive system with gluten. One of the highest rising allergies or sensitivities in modern Western societies is gluten/wheat intolerance. Over the years, many of my clients, both adults and children, have complained of feeling bloated after eating this kind of bread. A simple solution has been for them to eat traditionally made loaves instead.

During the process of traditional bread making the dough is allowed to ferment for long enough that naturally occurring beneficial bacteria have time to get to work making the bread more digestible, nutritious and delicious. With the Chorleywood Bread Process, however, the bread is made too quickly for these bacteria to have even a chance of getting to work. This results in a less digestible loaf as well as a loss of vitamins from the final loaf.

Compared to traditional bread making, the Chorleywood Bread Process uses many additional ingredients, a few of which don't legally have to be on the label. These additional ingredients include flour treatment agents, bleach, reducing agents, soya flour, emulsifiers, preservatives. Many of these commonly eaten loaves of bread will have very long ingredients lists while a more traditional loaf may have just three ingredients: flour, water, salt.

---

[5] https://fabflour.co.uk/fab-bread/the-chorleywood-bread-process-2/

Better Bread

A better bread to choose is a bread made by the traditional bread-making process. This is generally known today as a 'sourdough' bread, though sixty years ago it was just called 'bread'. You can also find some traditionally made rye breads too. Generally, if people are used to eating modern industrial bread then they will struggle to transition to real bread. That's because it has, as the name suggests, a slightly sour taste. Rye bread has quite a deep flavour and both of these traditional breads are far denser than their modern equivalents. They are chewier and tend to go off more quickly because they don't contain the preservatives and anti-fungal agents that keep Chorleywood breads from spoiling.

Depending on your family's preferences and the busyness of your schedule, these traditional breads may or may not be suitable. It might be that you decide to buy already sliced sourdough or rye bread or ask the bakery to slice the bread for you, then freeze it in portions and defrost as needed. That's one way around the spoiling issues. Furthermore, croutons from stale bread are great in soups. You'll find a recipe for those croutons on page 79.

Don't forget that pitta breads and flatbreads are also good options. Better flour and less yeast make for a more nutritious and digestible form of bread. Real foods tend to have fewer, more recognisable ingredients. An example below shows how many more ingredients you might find in a commercial wrap versus a traditional flatbread.

Finally, if this all sounds too complicated, or if you want simply

Traditional Flatbread	White Wrap
Wheat flour, water, oil, salt	Wheat flour, water, palm oil, humectant (vegetable glycerol), raising agents (disodium diphosphate, sodium hydrogen carbonate), sugar, emulsifier (mono- and diglycerides of fatty acids), citric acid, salt, preservative (calcium propionate), wheat starch, flour treatment agent (L-cysteine hydrochloride)

to avoid bread and go down the crispbread route, then there are many healthier wholefood options. Once again, look for minimal ingredients. Good examples tend to be:

- Rye crackers
- Oat crackers
- Seed-based crackers

Recipes

This chapter explores sandwich alternatives because bread is not a straightforward subject and more and more people are demanding variety in their lunches. You'll find these far more useful than a list of possible sandwich fillings that you could find all over the internet. Sandwich fillings don't help if you or your child don't like the taste or texture of 'real' bread.

Protein Pancakes

These pancakes can be eaten with savoury or sweet toppings. You can even sandwich two together and have some filling on the inside. Nut butters, yogurt and pâtés all work well with these slightly thicker (American-style) pancakes.

MAKES 4

15g ground flaxseeds
40g seeds (sunflower or pumpkin work well)
60g quinoa flakes or oats (gluten-free optional)
Pinch of salt
2 eggs, or 2 flax eggs (2 tbsp ground flaxseeds,
soaked in 6 tbsp warm water for 10 minutes)
200ml milk (dairy or non-dairy)
Coconut oil, butter or avocado oil, for frying

1   Grind the 2 kinds of seeds, quinoa flakes or oats and the salt in a food processor until you have a flour.
2   Add the eggs and milk and process again to form a batter.
3   Heat a small frying pan with a small dollop of oil or butter.
4   Add a large spoonful of batter. Flip when the pancake looks mostly cooked on one side, i.e. when bubbles appear across the surface. Cook the other side for 1 or 2 minutes.

Courgette, Sun-dried Tomato and Feta Bread

A deliciously moist, smooth vegetable loaf with great visual appeal. The tangy flavour of the feta shines through with bursts of sweetness from the sun-dried tomatoes with each and every mouthful.

MAKES 1 LOAF

A little olive oil, for greasing
125g plain gluten-free flour
1½ tsp baking powder
320g grated courgette,
squeeze out the liquid through muslin or a tea towel
30g chopped flat-leaf parsley
6 large eggs, beaten
200g feta, crumbled or roughly chopped
60g chopped sun-dried tomatoes

1   Preheat the oven to 190°C/Fan 170°C/Gas 5.
2   Grease and line (with greaseproof paper) a 2lb loaf tin.
3   In a large bowl, mix together the flour and baking powder. Stir in the courgette, parsley and eggs until combined. Gently mix in the feta and tomatoes.
4   Pour the batter into the prepared loaf tin.
5   Bake for 25 minutes, then cover in foil and bake for a further 25 minutes to prevent the top of the loaf burning.
6   Leave to cool then remove the bread from the tin. Slice and serve.

Savoury Oat Slice

Not everyone loves every vegetable, but the most common reason for not liking some vegetables is texture. When vegetables are grated and added to baked goods, even savoury bakes like this one, they are very often far better received. This slice is moist thanks to the vegetables and is deliciously cheesy too.

MAKES 10–12 PORTIONS

A little oil, for greasing
200g courgettes, grated
200g carrots, grated
1 medium onion, grated
2 large eggs, beaten, or 2 flax eggs
(2 tbsp ground flaxseeds soaked in 6 tbsp warm water for 10 minutes)
Good pinch of mixed herbs
200g flavoursome cheese, such as Parmesan or pecorino, grated
200g rolled oats

1   Preheat the oven to 200°C/Fan 180°C/Gas 6.
2   Line a shallow square baking tin of about 20 x 20cm or grease 10–12 sections of a 12-hole brownie tin.
3   Mix all the ingredients together well in a large bowl.
4   Place the mixture into the lined baking tin or greased brownie tin and cook for 25 minutes or until golden brown on the surface.
5   Cut into pieces and leave to cool before trying to remove the slices from the baking tin. If you're using a brownie tin, remove the individual pieces and leave to cool on a cooling rack.

Sweetcorn and Paprika Fritters

Sweetcorn is a popular vegetable. Those tasty little kernels add great, sweet flavour to this savoury fritter. These fritters can be served on their own, with a yogurt-style dip or low-sugar ketchup.

MAKES 4 LARGE OR 8 SMALL FRITTERS

230g tinned sweetcorn, drained weight
60g spelt flour or plain gluten-free flour
½ tsp baking powder
½ tsp salt
½ tsp sweet smoked paprika
1 extra large or 2 small eggs
2 tbsp olive oil or avocado oil

1 Put all the ingredients except the oil in a food processor and whizz to make a batter.
2 Heat a little of the oil in a frying pan and drop in heaped tablespoonfuls of the batter. Cook for about 90 seconds on each side. Repeat until you've used up all the batter.
3 Rest briefly on kitchen paper before leaving to cool.

Grain-free Pizza

This is a crispy-based pizza without any grains. It's incredibly filling and you can top it with your choice of vegetables and proteins to truly make it your own.

<u>SERVES 2</u>

170g ground almonds
85g arrowroot powder, plus extra for rolling
1 tsp baking powder
¾ tsp salt
½ tsp dried oregano
1 large egg
25g coconut oil, melted
40ml almond milk
3 tbsp passata
1 large portobello mushroom, thinly sliced
6–8 cherry tomatoes, halved
5 slices of bresaola or Parma ham, roughly torn
1 tsp olive oil
Salt and pepper
Rocket leaves, to serve

1   Preheat the oven to 200°C/Fan 180°C/Gas 6.
2   Stir together the almonds, arrowroot, baking powder, salt and dried oregano in a large bowl.
3   Whisk together the egg, oil and milk in a small bowl.
4   Combine the egg mix and the almond mix gradually to form a stiff dough.
5   Roll the dough out on greaseproof paper (this is going to go directly on to your baking sheet, so make sure it will fit) to about ½ cm thick. Use a little extra arrowroot powder to avoid sticking.
6   Place the greaseproof paper on to your baking sheet and bake for 10 minutes.

7   Next, increase the temperature to 220°C/Fan 200°C/Gas 7. Using a second baking sheet on top of the first, carefully turn the pizza base over and bake the other side for another 6 minutes (check that the base is cooked in the middle).

8   Spread the passata over the base, then add the mushroom slices, cherry tomato halves, bresaola or Parma ham. Drizzle over the olive oil and add a little seasoning. Bake for 5–10 more minutes, until the tomatoes and mushrooms are no longer raw. Serve hot with rocket leaves sprinkled over the top.

Crustless Quiche Lorraine

Salty bacon and nutty Gruyère cheese combine to please the palate. This quiche is made without the traditional crust because a) it's so tasty it doesn't need a crust and b) some people are simply better off without the crust.

SERVES 4

6 slices of back bacon
1 tsp olive oil, plus extra for greasing
1 onion, diced
2 garlic cloves, crushed
6 large eggs
175ml milk
200g Gruyère cheese, grated

1   Preheat the oven to 200°C/Fan 180°C/Gas 6.
2   Cook the bacon in the oil in a frying pan over a medium heat until crispy. Remove from the pan, chop or slice and leave to cool.
3   Add the onion to the fat left in the pan. Cook for 5 minutes, until transparent.
4   Add in the garlic. Sauté for 30 seconds. Remove from the heat and leave to cool.
5   In a large bowl, whisk together the eggs and milk. Stir in the cheese, bacon and cooked onions with garlic.
6   Grease and line a 25 x 15cm baking tin. Pour the mixture into the prepared tin.
7   Bake for 30 minutes or until the egg mixture has set. You can check this with a cocktail stick.
8   Cool completely before slicing and serving in lunches.

Courgette Pesto Mini Quiches

Few of us have a lot of time on our hands, so a recipe that allows you to mix, pour and bake just three ingredients is one to remember. This is one to make and bake over and over.

½ tsp olive oil, for greasing (unless using a non-stick muffin tin)
½ a medium courgette, very thinly sliced using a vegetable peeler
2 large eggs
1 tbsp red pesto
Salt and pepper

1 Preheat the oven to 200°C/Fan 180°C/Gas 6.
2 Grease 2 holes of a deep muffin tin with oil using a pastry brush. If you are using a non-stick muffin tin, there is no need to do this.
3 Line each hole with thinly sliced courgette
4 Whisk the egg and pesto together in a bowl. Season with a little salt and pepper.
5 Pour the egg and pesto mixture into the muffin holes.
6 Bake for 15–20 minutes. Leave to cool a little before removing the quiches from the tin. Cool completely before adding to your packed lunch.

Grain-free Bread

This moist bread works as a brilliant sandwich bread. It's mighty filling so you'll need only a few thin slices to replace normal, commercial bread slices.

100g nuts of your choice (walnuts, cashews, almonds all work well)
40g ground flaxseeds
30g coconut flour
1 tsp bicarbonate of soda
½ tsp salt
40g melted coconut oil
1 tbsp raw honey
1 tsp apple cider vinegar
4 extra large eggs (80g) or 6–7 smaller eggs

1 Preheat the oven to 200°C/Fan 180°C/Gas 6.
2 Use a food processor to grind the nuts and seeds until they have a fine consistency like flour. Add the coconut flour, bicarbonate of soda and the salt and stir.
3 Add the coconut oil, honey, vinegar and eggs, then stir again.
4 Pour the mixture into a greased, lined bread tin and bake for 40 minutes. Check it is cooked through by inserting a toothpick into the centre of the bread. Leave to cool before removing it from the tin.

Gluten-free Loaf

I first tasted this bread when it was prepared for me by a chef called Adrian Foster from our local biodynamic farm, Waltham Place. He'd found this recipe at www.thebreadkitchen.com. All I've done is change the vegetable oil to olive oil and used apple cider vinegar instead of any other kind. It's a delicious, naturally gluten-free bread. It doesn't last long before it starts to crumble but that's because it doesn't contain lots of preservatives. Eat it quick!

MAKES 1 LOAF

A little extra olive oil, for greasing
450g buckwheat flour
2 tsp dried yeast
1 tsp salt
2 tsp sugar or honey
290ml warm water
2 tbsp extra virgin olive oil
1 tsp apple cider vinegar
2 eggs

1   Preheat the oven to 220°C/Fan 200°C/Gas 7.
2   Grease and line a 2lb loaf tin with greaseproof paper.
3   Place all the dry ingredients in a bowl and mix well.
4   Combine all the wet ingredients in a bowl and mix well.
5   Add the wet ingredients to the dry ingredients. Mix very well with the handle of a wooden spoon to form a thick batter that drops sluggishly off the spoon.
6   Pour the batter into the prepared loaf tin and allow it to prove in a warm place until the dough just fills the tin. Do not over-prove or the loaf will collapse during cooking.
7   Bake for about 25–30 minutes.
8   Rest the loaf in the tin for 10 minutes before turning it out to cool on a wire rack.

Sweet Potato Crust Quiche

The sweet potato crust of this quiche contrasts deliciously with the creamy spinach and cheese filling. What's more, there are vegetables in both the crust and the filling so it's a win-win nutritionally. This recipe has been adapted from an original by Little Cooks Co, who provide healthy cooking kits for kids.

SERVES 8

435g sweet potato, grated
60g Cheddar cheese
1 egg
A little olive oil, for greasing
Salt and pepper

Quiche filling
120g frozen spinach (frozen weight), defrosted
5 eggs
75g Cheddar cheese
100ml cream

1   Preheat the oven to 190°C/Fan 170°C/Gas 5.
2   Squeeze the grated potato through a muslin to remove the excess liquid.
3   Mix the sweet potato together with the cheese, egg and seasoning.
4   Grease and line a 25 x 15cm baking tin with greaseproof paper.
5   Push the 'dough' into the base of the tin to make the quiche base. Then bake for 20 minutes.
6   In another bowl, mix all the filling ingredients together. Add these to the pre-baked quiche base and bake for another 20 minutes. Remove and cover the quiche with foil to prevent the crust from burning and cook for another 20 minutes, until the egg is cooked through. Cool then serve.

Frittata

This is such an adaptable recipe. Simply whisk eggs and cheese together then pour over the vegetables of your choice and bake. How easy is that? More importantly, how flexible is that?

SERVES 2

2 tsp olive oil, for greasing
4 extra large eggs (80g each)
50ml cream
50g Cheddar cheese, grated
1 tbsp chopped fresh parsley
10 cherry tomatoes, halved
1 pepper, finely chopped
50g frozen peas, defrosted
Salt and pepper

1 Preheat the oven to 200°C/Fan 180°C/Gas 6.
2 Grease and line a 20 x 20cm ovenproof dish with greaseproof paper.
3 Whisk the eggs, cream and cheese together in a large bowl. Add the parsley and season.
4 Place the vegetables into the ovenproof dish. Then pour the egg and cheese mixture over the vegetables.
5 Cook in the oven for 20 minutes until the frittata is golden brown and set.
6 Leave to cool before removing and serve cold in your lunchbox.

Chestnut Pancakes

These fully grain-free, gluten-free, slightly sweet and nutty-tasting pancakes are fantastic served with a variety of savoury fillings, especially leftover cooked vegetables. They taste delicious with cheese and mushrooms, but equally they could be folded up and served with soup or even a bean casserole, stew or chilli.

MAKES 4 PANCAKES

100g chestnut flour
125ml milk (dairy-free optional)
1 egg
1½ tsp butter, olive oil or coconut oil, plus a little extra for cooking

1   Blend all the ingredients together with 125ml of water, in a food processor or bowl.
2   Add a little extra oil or butter to a crêpe pan.
3   Add 2 dessertspoonfuls of the batter (about 90–100ml) to the pan. Allow the pancake to cook on the underside until the surface no longer appears wet.
4   Turn the pancake over and cook the other side. Repeat with the remaining butter.
5   Fill with your chosen ingredients and/or fold over. Serve in your lunchbox.

Cottage Cheese Pancakes

These pancakes are light and fluffy. There's flexibility in terms of what you serve them with – savoury or sweet. Cold meats and lettuce are delicious. Fruits, such as mixed berries, are yum too. The recipe makes four pancakes so you could easily sandwich ingredients between two pancakes for two people's lunches.

MAKES 4 PANCAKES

3 eggs
50g rolled oats, ground to a flour
100g cottage cheese
½ tsp olive oil

1   Mix all the ingredients, except the oil, together in a food processor or simply mix together well in a bowl.
2   Add a drizzle of oil to a crêpe pan.
3   Heat the oil then add a quarter of the batter.
4   Cook until the batter starts to bubble then turn the pancake over and cook on the other side. Repeat until you have used up all the batter.

Buckwheat Blinis

These little pancakes are a great 'paddle' – for want of a better word!
– for dips and cream cheese. They're also gluten-free as buckwheat
is part of the same family as rhubarb and sorrel.

MAKES 8–10 BLINIS

1 tbsp olive oil, for frying
1 egg
90g buckwheat flour
1 tsp baking powder
150ml milk (non-dairy milk optional)

1   Heat the oil in a wide frying pan.
2   Whisk the egg in a large mixing bowl. Add the flour, baking
    powder and milk, then stir until evenly mixed, to form a batter.
3   Dollop spoonfuls of the batter into the hot oil, allowing a little
    room at the edges for the batter to spread. Once you see large
    bubbles form in the pancake, turn it over and cook on the other
    side.
4   Remove from the pan and briefly lay on kitchen paper to
    remove any excess fat. Repeat until you have used up all the
    batter.
5   Serve with hummus, cream cheese and dips.

Moroccan Chickpea Patties

A taste of Northern Africa. These patties are delicious paired
with something yogurt-based like tzatziki or simply Greek yogurt
itself in the lunchbox. These are also great with a cucumber
dill salad (p.69).

MAKES 4 PATTIES

1 x 400g tin of chickpeas, rinsed and drained
1 garlic clove, minced
1 egg
1 tbsp plain flour or plain gluten-free flour
2 tsp harissa paste
1 tsp ground cumin
1 tbsp chopped mint
1 tbsp chopped parsley
1 tbsp olive oil, for frying

1   In a food processor, combine all the ingredients except the oil.
2   Heat the oil in a large frying pan.
3   Add 4 large spoonfuls of batter to the pan with spaces in
    between each. Pat down the batter with the back of the spoon.
4   Turn the pancakes over after about 3–4 minutes. Cook on the
    other side. Cool, then serve in lunchboxes.

Smoked Trout and Cheese Muffins

Salty smoked trout and cheese combine in these grain-free, protein-rich muffins. They're jam-packed full of flavour.

MAKES 4 MUFFINS

Olive oil, for greasing
4 eggs
100g smoked trout, thinly sliced
2 tbsp grated cheese (pecorino, Cheddar, Gruyère)
A pinch of salt (leave this out if using mature or saltier cheese)
2 spring onions, thinly sliced on the diagonal

1   Preheat the oven to 200°C/Fan 180°C/Gas 6.
2   Grease 4 muffin holes in a muffin tin with a little oil.
3   Mix together the eggs, trout, cheese and salt in a bowl.
4   Pour the mixture into the 4 greased muffin holes. Bake for
    20 minutes or until the muffins are firm and cooked through.
5   Leave to cool then remove from the muffin tin.

5 A Simple Way to 10-a-Day

Why Vegetables Need a Marketing Budget

Vegetables are not only hugely varied in colour, taste and texture, they're also a great source of fibre, vitamins, minerals and phytonutrients. Yet they have it tough. They don't have glitzy ad campaigns. They don't have huge marketing budgets spent on raising people's awareness of their extensive health benefits. How are they supposed to come out on top when the overwhelming message is that manufactured foods with health claims plastered all over the packaging are the foods we should be focusing our attention and both pester and buying power on?

Governments in countries all over the world have struggled to raise awareness of the need to eat vegetables as part of a balanced diet. The stats consistently show that few people eat enough vegetables each day. Yet, it is hard to make changes to our behaviour without sufficient reason to do so or if the change does not appear realistically achievable. The idea behind this chapter is to explain why eating vegetables and fruit is important but also to show how easy it can be to achieve not just five-a-day but even ten.

Why are Vegetables and Fruit So Good for Us?

We hear so much about whether we should or shouldn't be eating food from different food groups. In amongst that noise from various media sources and the diet fads vying for our attention, the one thing that remains constant is the healthiness of eating vegetables. Likewise with fruit. Their value in terms of contributing to longevity and well-being is undisputed. Further evidence of this is the focus on vegetables consistent amongst the Blue Zones. These are areas of the world in which people live exceptionally long lives. Studies have found that what these people eat contributes to this longevity and vegetables and fruit are a key component.

Complex Carbohydrates

One of the reasons vegetables come so highly recommended is that the vast majority are classed as what is known as 'complex carbohydrates'. That means they release energy more slowly into the body than other foods because they break down into glucose, the body's preferred energy source, much more slowly than other foods. We find ourselves surrounded by fast food, junk food and processed food – foods that are designed by manufacturers not only to biologically make us crave more but also to cause spikes in our blood glucose levels followed by subsequent blood glucose lows. Complex carbohydrates, and vegetables in particular, are a welcome reprieve from this, proving that nature really does know best. Vegetables are a necessary part of a balanced diet, not least because they help us sustain consistent energy levels over time.

Fibre

Vegetables and fruit are also good sources of fibre. Few of us get sufficient fibre in our diets currently. In fact, on average adults consume 18g of fibre per day compared to the recommended UK government guidelines of 30g per day[6]. While children's targets are slightly lower, these are not currently being reached either. On average, children under sixteen years of age are only getting 15g or less fibre per day. Children's fibre intake targets are as follows:

2–5 years: 15g per day
5–11 years: 20g per day
11–16 years: 25g per day

Simply increasing our intake of vegetables and fruit could go a long way to helping improve our fibre consumption. A medium apple, a stalk of broccoli and a medium-sized carrot contain about 3g of fibre each. That's 9g of fibre alone. Eating fruit and vegetables throughout the day makes it easy for fibre levels to tot up.

Fibre also has a way of slowing down the release of carbohydrates and thus glucose into the body. This means we are less likely to experience fluctuations in our performance, mood and appetite when consuming a fibre-rich diet. Fibre also allows us to feel fuller for longer, which means we are less likely to snack in between meals and we are also likely to make better food choices when we get to mealtimes. That's because we are less attracted to the quickest, and often least healthy, option in order to satiate our hunger and boost our blood glucose levels.

[6] https://www.nhs.uk/live-well/eat-well/how-to-get-more-fibre-into-your-diet/

Added to that, a fibre-rich diet can help increase the good bacteria in the gut. Fibre provides a food source for 'friendly' gut bacteria, helping them to increase and produce substances which are thought to be protective to the lining of the gut. It is a little-known fact that one of the reasons for increased sensitivity to foods is that the lining of the gut has become compromised. A low-fibre diet is one of the factors that contributes to this, but it is easily rectified. So, eating more vegetables and fruit could help improve overall energy levels and even contribute to improved digestion and absorption of nutrients.

Antioxidants

Vegetables and fruit are sources of antioxidants. You could view antioxidants as an army. They help protect us by preventing damage to our body tissues. These compounds found in vegetables and fruit are believed to be of vital importance in preventing major degenerative diseases, such as cancer, heart disease and strokes, and also in boosting our immune system and preventing sports-related injuries.

As a rule of thumb the more brightly or deeply coloured a vegetable, the more antioxidants it contains. Let's take lettuce as an example. While most lettuces are green, the darker green leaves are more nutritious and contain more antioxidants than lighter green leaves. On a scale of iceberg, which is the least nutritious, to watercress, the most nutritious, you can judge how antioxidant-rich and nutrient-dense your choices might be.

Variety

You only have to walk into a greengrocer or the fresh produce section of your local supermarket to realise that there is a huge variety of fresh vegetables and fruit for us to choose from. Yet, typically, most of us get stuck in a rut. We tend to stick to what we know and end up eating the same four to eight vegetables and fruit. Some of this is due to familiarity and what we know how to cook or prepare, or in the case of children what we know will get eaten (I call this 'the broccoli, peas and carrots trap'), but there's a whole rainbow of variety out there. Try to choose at least one vegetable or fruit from every colour grouping per day. While eating fruit seems to be easier than eating vegetables for many, perhaps owing to the fact that it is sweet, try to aim for a ratio of 3:1 vegetables to fruit for a better mix of nutrients without overloading the body with sugar.

Red	Green	Blue/Purple	White	Yellow-Orange
Apples	Spinach	Blueberries	Garlic	Apricots
Blood Orange	Celery	Blackberries	Ginger	Butternut Squash
Red Cabbage	Broccoli	Beetroot	Cauliflower	Carrots
Cranberries	Green Peppers	Plums	Mushrooms	Grapefruit
Cherries	Brussels Sprouts	Aubergine	Onions	Canteloupe
Pomegranates	Green Beans	Purple Carrots	Shallots	Lemons
Radishes	Cucumber	Figs	Turnips	Oranges
Red Peppers	Leafy Greens	Purple Asparagus	Pears	Mangoes
Raspberries	Asparagus	Purple Broccoli	Yam	Papayas
Strawberries	Avocado	Black Grapes	White Peaches	Pumpkin
Tomatoes	Kiwi	Elderberries	Coconut	Sweet Potatoes
Red Grapes	Courgette	Red Cabbage	Lychees	Tangerines
Red Apples	Green Apples	Purple Cauliflower	Jerusalem Artichokes	
Pineapple				

How to Eat More Vegetables and Fruit

In this chapter, I'll show how easily vegetables and fruits can be used and served. But how do you reach ten portions a day? First, you'll need to know what constitutes a portion by age, and this table can help with that:

	1–4 years	5–7 years	8–11 years	12+
Banana	½ small	½ small	1 small	1 large
Broccoli	1 floret	2 florets	3 florets	4 florets
Raisins	1 tbsp	2 tbsp	2 tbsp	Handful
Grated carrot	1 tbsp	1 tbsp	2 tbsp	3 tbsp
Cherry tomatoes	2	3	4	5
Satsuma	1	1	1–2	2
Cooked pulses	¼ cup	½ cup	¾ cup	1 cup
Berries	1–2 tbsp	2 tbsp	3 tbsp	4 tbsp
Cooked veg e.g. beans	1–2 tbsp	2 tbsp	2–3 tbsp	3–4 tbsp
Cucumber	2–3 slices	3–4 slices	4–6 slices	6 slices
Dried apricots	3	4	6	6–8
Grapes	8	10	12	15
Kiwi fruit	1	2	2	2
Apple/orange/pear	1–2	1 medium	1 med. – 1 large	1 large
Melon	25g	50g	50g	100g
Sweetcorn kernels	1 tbsp	2 tbsp	2 tbsp	3 tbsp

Easy Ways to Include Vegetables in a Lunchbox

There are many ways to include vegetables in a lunchbox. Most of us tend to get caught in the habitual trap of serving vegetables as batons or in a salad. The possibilities are numerous though.

Served:	Vegetable	Used how?
Batons	Pepper	With dips
	Carrot	Just as they are
	Celery	
	Cucumber	
	Courgette	
	Sugar snap peas	
	Baby corn	
Grated	Carrot	Sandwiches
	Beetroot	Salads
	Courgette	Muffins
	Cucumber	Just as they are
Leaves	Spinach	Frittatas
	Kale	Salads
		Curries
Vegetable noodles	Cucumber	In place of pasta
	Carrot	In salads
	Butternut squash	Just as they are
Frozen	Peas	Just as they are – they defrost
	Sweetcorn	perfectly by lunchtime
Raw florets	Broccoli	As a crunchy accompaniment to a dip
	Cauliflower	Grated in salads
		Just as they are
Cooked	Root vegetables	Soups
	Cruciferous vegetables	Curries
	Non-starchy vegetables	Stews
	Dark green leafy vegetables	Casseroles

Building a Salad

One of the most practical ways to increase vegetable and fruit consumption is to build a layered salad to take to work or school in a jar – either glass or plastic. All you do is layer up the salad using the simple, easy-to-follow steps that follow. When you're ready for lunch simply open the separate container of dressing, pour it into the jar, replace the jar lid and shake. All that's left to do is remove the lid and tuck in!

Here is the simple formula to help you decide what should go into your jar.

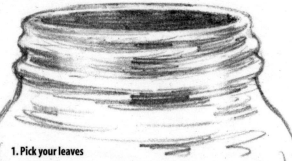

1. Pick your leaves

As a rule of thumb the most nutritious leaves are the darkest ones – for example rocket, watercress, spinach and kale – and the least nutritious are the lightest coloured leaves, such as iceberg. To begin with, choose whatever you or your child like best.

2. Pick your vegetables/fruit

There are lots of choices. Some delicious vegetable and fruit choices for salads include, but are not limited to, cucumbers, carrots, courgettes, broccoli, avocados, celery, radishes, sugar snap peas, tomatoes, cauliflowers, apples, pears, figs, grapes, apricots.

3. Add your protein

From animal proteins, such as cold cooked meats (chicken, turkey, ham, beef) through to fish (salmon, sardines, tuna, mackerel) to eggs and cheese, and vegetable proteins, such as tofu/tempeh, beans and pulses, there's quite a range to choose from.

4. Add some crunch

Salads are even more enjoyable when they have some texture. Try seeds, nuts, crispy bacon or croutons.

5. A handful of carbs

Add some starchy vegetables, such as sweet potato, new potatoes, butternut squash, beetroot, or noodles, rice, pasta.

6. Dressing

There are many shop-bought dressings that are made from simple, recognisable ingredients. If you do want to make your own choose roughly 120ml of oil to 60ml of vinegar, e.g. apple cider, balsamic, red wine or white wine, or an acidic ingredient, e.g. lime juice, lemon juice, grapefruit juice (or a combination of both), then add some flavour like honey, mustard, soy sauce/tamari, ginger, herbs, tahini, nut butter.

Building Your Own Pot Noodle

At one stage or another most of us will have tried or been tempted by the ease of a pot noodle. We know they're not the best meal

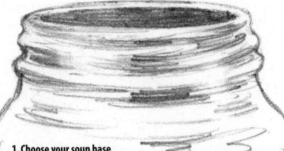

1. Choose your soup base

You will need 1–3 teaspoons of miso soup paste, bouillon, curry paste (Thai, Chinese or Indian are all options) or chipotle paste.

2. Choose your vegetables

You will need about 100g of vegetables. Make sure you stick with vegetables that can be eaten raw. For firmer vegetables, such as carrots, cabbage, leeks, larger mushrooms, either grate the vegetables on the large holes of a box grater or cut them into thin matchsticks.

Frozen vegetables, such as peas or corn, can be added directly from the freezer, though if you plan on cooking the pots immediately, it's best to thaw them under the tap first so that you don't lose too much heat when you add your boiling water.

3. Add some protein

Such as tofu, tempeh, cooked meats, cooked eggs, finely chopped jerky/biltong.

4. Add your noodles

The best options are wok-ready noodles sold in the fresh vegetable section of the supermarket or vermicelli rice noodles. However, you can also use leftover cooked pasta (spaghetti or linguine) in these pots, too.

5. Add hot water (only at lunchtime!)

When you're ready for lunch, add 280ml of hot water. Stir the contents of the jar. Replace the lid then leave for five minutes.

6. Stir in some extra flavour

For added taste, why not stir in some soy sauce/tamari, herbs, chilli sauce, lemon or lime juice, coconut cream, or any other flavours you enjoy.

nutritionally, but we are attracted by the warm, salty flavours and the allure of something so convenient during the busy lunchtime period. Another use for the glass jar is to take something to work (providing there is a kettle) and create a hot meal to enjoy after just five minutes of steeping – your very own pot noodle. Of course, you must ensure that your glass jar is heatproof. It's worth investing in a better-quality one for this reason.

Recipes

This chapter celebrates vegetables and fruit, showcasing multiple ways to enjoy them in your packed lunches.

Baked Vegetable Frittata

Eggs, cheese and vegetables baked in a pan. A great way to use up leftover cooked vegetables or any vegetables that are still in the fridge at the end of the week.

SERVES 2–4

1 medium courgette, sliced into 5 x 2cm batons
2 large flat mushrooms, diced
½ tsp olive oil
8 eggs, beaten
40g pecorino or Parmesan, grated
2 tbsp chopped fresh flat-leaf parsley
Black pepper

1   Preheat the oven to 200°C/Fan 180°C/Gas 6.
2   Lay all the vegetables in a small roasting tin, about 30 x 15cm.
3   Drizzle over the oil and sprinkle with salt. Bake for 15 minutes, tossing once while cooking.
4   Beat the eggs and the cheese together and add the parsley and a good twist of black pepper.
5   Pour this over the cooked vegetables and bake for another 15 minutes or until the egg is completely set.
6   Cool and slice then serve or serve warm in a warmed flask (see The Value of Insulated Flasks on p.96 for how to warm your flask).

Roasted Cauliflower and Bacon

When these two ingredients are roasted and combined it's like a flavour explosion. This combination could be served cold, but ideally hot for lunch. Serve in an insulated flask for the hot option.

250g cauliflower, cut into small florets
2 garlic cloves, thinly sliced
100g free range or organic unsmoked lardons or bacon pieces
1 tsp olive oil
Sea salt and freshly ground black pepper

1   Preheat the oven to 200°C/Fan 180°C/Gas 6.
2   Toss together the cauliflower, garlic, bacon and olive oil on a baking sheet.
3   Roast for 35–45 minutes until the bacon is cooked and the cauliflower is both cooked and starting to crisp around the edges.
4   Season with salt and pepper to taste.
5   Cool or place in insulated flasks immediately.

Pan-fried Vegetable Quinoa

Quinoa is what is known as a pseudo-grain. It can be eaten in the same dishes as you might find couscous, bulgur wheat or even rice. It's a slow-release carbohydrate that's delicious when perfectly cooked and paired with sweet, gently sautéed vegetables.

SERVES 2–4

1 tbsp olive oil or avocado oil
1 courgette, chopped into 2cm cubes
1 yellow pepper, chopped into two 2cm squares
10 cherry tomatoes, halved
200g cooked quinoa (to make this you'll need about 120g quinoa and about 340ml water plus some salt – bring this to the boil then simmer gently until the quinoa is soft)
1 tbsp chopped fresh herbs (flat-leaf parsley and oregano/marjoram work well)
Salt and pepper

1   Heat 1 teaspoon of the oil in a small frying pan. Add the vegetables and sauté them for about 10 minutes until soft.
2   Stir in the cooked quinoa and the rest of the oil, then season to taste. Finally, stir in the fresh herbs.
3   Leave to cool and serve on its own or as part of a salad.

Butternut Squash Falafels

Falafels provide a substantial non-meat alternative in a lunchbox. These falafels use the natural sweetness of roasted butternut squash to give both great flavour and texture. The falafel mixture needs to be prepared 24 hours before cooking.

SERVES 4–6

400g cooked butternut squash (approximately 1 squash peeled, deseeded and roasted until soft, or you can bake the squash whole, then peel and use the flesh)
100g tinned chickpeas, rinsed
2 tbsp gram flour
½ tsp ground coriander
1 tsp ground cumin
Juice of ¼ lemon
2 tbsp olive oil or avocado oil

1   Put all ingredients except the oil into a food processor and whizz to combine to form a smooth, thick paste.
2   Leave in the fridge for 24 hours.
3   Mould the mixture into small falafel balls.
4   Heat the oil in a frying pan.
5   Lightly fry the falafels until crispy on the outside but fluffy and sweet on the inside.
6   Drain using a piece of kitchen paper on a plate.
7   Serve cooled in a lunchbox alongside vegetables or a salad.

Simple Tricolore Salad

We eat with our eyes, so the saying goes. This salad combines three distinct colours – white, red and green. It's visually appealing, easy to make and easy to eat too.

SERVES 1–2

6 mozzarella balls
6 cherry tomatoes, halved
6 cucumber cubes (about the same size as the tomato halves)
2 tsp green pesto (optional)

1   Combine the mozzarella and vegetables in a small container with a lid. You could stir 2 teaspoons of green pesto into this little salad if you like. It brings the ingredients together nicely.

Sweet Potato and Bean Cakes

This recipe makes a really moist and delicious bean burger,
seasoned with the natural flavours of Mexico. The patties need to be
prepared the night before you want to cook them.

MAKES ABOUT 10 PATTIES

1 x 200g cooked sweet potato (weight without skin)
1 x 400g tin of pinto beans, drained and rinsed
1 tsp chipotle paste
3 tbsp plain flour or plain gluten-free flour, plus a little extra for dusting
2 tbsp chopped fresh coriander
2 tbsp olive oil

1   Combine all the ingredients, except the oil, in a food processor.
2   Using a little extra flour, shape the mixture into about 10
    patties. Lay these flat on a baking sheet and refrigerate
    overnight.
3   The following morning, heat the oil in a large pan. Add half the
    patties to the pan.
4   Cook on one side then turn over. You should end up cooking the
    patties for about 5 minutes in total. They are a little fiddly so be
    careful when turning.
5   Cook the second batch.
6   Serve with some mayonnaise or yogurt dip.

Carrot and Raisin Salad

This simple salad combines some great flavours of the Middle East. It's a delicious salad to have with hummus and/or baked pitta chips (see p.139).

(see p.139)

SERVES 1–2

---

1 large carrot or 2 small
20g raisins
20g flaked almonds (optional)
1 tsp olive oil
¼ tsp balsamic vinegar
Salt and pepper

1   Grate the carrot by hand.
2   Add the raisins and flaked almonds.
3   Then add the olive oil and balsamic vinegar. Mix well.
4   Add a twist of salt and pepper and serve.

Carrot and Courgette 'Spaghetti' with Avocado Pesto

You don't need a spiraliser to create vegetable spaghetti. A julienne peeler will do. This recipe uses vegetable noodles in place of wheat-based noodles. Along with the creamy avocado-based pesto, this is a great dish for reaching your ten-a-day target. If vegetable spaghetti is not your thing then, forego that element but don't forego the pesto. It's too delicious and creamy not to try it on pasta or a sandwich.

SERVES 2

1 medium courgette
1 large carrot
¼ tsp olive oil, for sautéing, and 2 tbsp for the pesto
20g pack of fresh basil, washed and patted dry
1 medium avocado (about 100g), peeled and destoned
20g toasted pine nuts
1 tbsp lemon juice
50g Emmental cheese, grated
1 garlic clove, crushed
3 sun-dried tomatoes, thinly sliced (optional)

1   Use a julienne peeler or spiraliser to create spaghetti with the courgette and carrot.
2   Heat the ¼ teaspoon of olive oil in a medium-sized frying pan and sauté the vegetables for a couple of minutes. Set aside.
3   In a food processor, combine the basil, avocado, pine nuts, lemon juice, cheese and garlic. Add the olive oil and process again.
4   Stir the pesto into the cooked vegetables strands (or cooked pasta if preferred) while they are still warm to allow the pesto to melt into the vegetable spaghetti or pasta. Stir in the sun-dried tomatoes, if using. Serve warm by transporting the spaghetti in an insulated flask.

Roasted Mediterranean-style Feta

This is a bit of a cheat meal. However, it's well worth the indulgence for the reward of great flavour and a taste of the Mediterranean.

½ x 280g jar of grilled peppers antipasti
½ x 280g jar of grilled aubergine antipasti
½ x 280g jar of grilled courgette antipasti
200g feta, cubed
Juice and zest of ½ lemon
Extra virgin olive oil, for drizzling (optional)

1 Preheat the oven to 200°C/Fan 180°C/Gas 6.
2 Drain the antipasti and feta.
3 Toss the antipasti and feta together in a small roasting tin and squeeze over the lemon juice, add the zest and stir. There should be enough oil from the antipasti but if not drizzle over some extra virgin olive oil before roasting.
4 Roast for 15 minutes. Place each portion into a flask. Best served warm.

Cinnamon-toasted Butternut Squash

Some vegetables can get a bit boring if prepared and served in the same way each time. Butternut squash lends itself to roasting and therefore sweetening up. Its texture and flavour combine well with cinnamon for a delicious vegetable option that can be eaten on its own or as part of a salad.

SERVES 4–6 (AS A VEGETABLE PORTION)

½ a medium-sized butternut squash, chopped into 2–3cm cubes
¼–½ tsp ground cinnamon (depending on preference)
1½ tsp of olive oil
Salt

1   Preheat the oven to 200°C/Fan 180°C/Gas 6.
2   Place the butternut squash in a roasting pan.
3   Season with salt and sprinkle with the cinnamon and add the olive oil.
4   Roast in the preheated oven for 30–35 minutes until soft.

Carrot and Spice Chickpea or Yellow Pea Pancakes

Vegetables appear in pancakes all over the world. It's not uncommon and so neither should it be uncommon in our packed lunches. Here we bring together some delicious Asian flavours in a moist and satisfying pancake. This can be served as is but it also goes well with yogurt and Asian pickles. You could even combine it with one of the curries in the Hot Meals chapter or a dip.

MAKES 4–5 PANCAKES

40g rice flour
100g chickpea or yellow pea flour
½ tsp bicarbonate of soda
½ tsp garam masala
¼ tsp ground cumin
tsp ground turmeric
¼ tsp salt
1 medium carrot, grated
1 large egg, beaten
Olive oil, for frying

1 Mix together the flours, bicarbonate of soda, spices and salt in a bowl.
2 Add the grated carrot to the flour mix then add 200–250ml of water and the egg to make a thick cream consistency.
3 Heat ½ teaspoon of olive oil in a frying pan.
4 Add a dollop of the batter (about a dessertspoonful).
5 You'll know when to flip the pancake because small bubbles will appear on the surface. Cook on the other side for a few minutes.
6 Remove the pancake from the pan and leave to cool. Continue until all the batter has been used.
7 Serve in your lunchbox with a curry or some yogurt and pickles.

Mexican Tuna Nachos/Pitta Chips

This is a Mexican-themed lunchtime dip served with salted tortilla chips or baked pitta chips. It makes a change from the simple tuna mayo sandwich.

SERVES 6–8

1 x 400g tin of pinto beans, drained and mashed with the back of a fork or processed using a food processor to a paste
1 x 110g tin of tuna in olive oil (undrained)
1 yellow pepper, finely diced
100g mild salsa
Plain salted tortilla chips (shop-bought) or pitta chips (either shop-bought or home-made – see p.139)
3 tbsp grated Cheddar cheese

1   Simply mix the pinto beans, tuna, yellow pepper and salsa together in a bowl or food processor.
2   Serve the dip in a transportable container with the cheese scattered over each portion.
3   Serve the tortilla chips (nachos) or pitta chips alongside.

Cucumber Dill Salad

Cucumber is lovely but some complain that it's lacking in flavour.
Add the powerful flavours of lemon, dill and salt with creamy yogurt
and you'll be transported to a Greek taverna in the summertime.

SERVES 2–4

1 whole ridged cucumber, halved lengthways and thinly sliced across
200g yogurt
1½ tbsp chopped fresh dill
1 tbsp lemon juice
Salt

1   In a medium bowl, mix the ingredients together. Season to
     taste.
2   Cover and leave to cool for at least 4 hours or overnight before
     serving.

Sweet Potato Fingers

Who doesn't like chips? We all know that we can't eat chips all the
time. Sweet potato fingers though . . . they're another matter
entirely. Soft and sweet on the inside, crispy on the outside. Yum!

MAKES ABOUT 20 FINGERS

400g sweet potatoes, scrubbed and cut into fingers (leave the skin on)
20g olive oil
¼ tsp salt
¼ tsp sweet smoked paprika
15g dried breadcrumbs (can choose gluten-free)

1   Heat the oven to 200°C/Fan 180°C/Gas 6.
2   Toss the sweet potatoes with the oil, salt, paprika and
    breadcrumbs in a large bowl, massaging them well to coat.
3   Spread the sweet potato out on 2 baking trays, then roast for
    30–35 minutes until tender on the inside and crisp on the
    outside. Turn the potatoes halfway so that the fingers cook
    evenly.

Corn on the Cob

While we probably all know how to prepare corn on the cob – in simple terms, boil or steam until you can smell the distinct aroma of buttery sweetcorn – there are lots of different ways to serve it.

1 HALF COB PER PERSON FOR LUNCH

Butter, garlic butter or mayonnaise, to serve

1   This is just one way to do it: simply put your corn on the cobs into a pot of boiling, salted water.
2   Boil until you can smell the distinct aroma. The corn should become brighter yellow in colour too.
3   Remove from the pot and drain. Leave to cool before serving in your packed lunch. Or transport hot in a flask. They can be smothered in a coating of your choice.

Traffic Light Kebabs

This is a colourful way to enjoy a variety of popular fruits.

SERVES 1–2

2 ripe kiwi fruit
½ mango
¼ pineapple
8 strawberries

1   Chop the kiwi, mango and pineapple into chunks the same size as the strawberries.
2   Push these on to cocktail sticks or reusable straws in the order they would appear on a traffic light: red (strawberry), amber (mango and pineapple) and green (kiwi).
3   Pop into your lunchbox.

Tropical Fruit Salad

These deliciously sweet fruits work so well together in a sweet fruit salad. As a combination of the sweetest fruits, also served with honey, yogurt works well alongside.

1 pineapple
1 mango
½ a cantaloupe melon
1 tbsp honey (or less if your fruit is very ripe)
½ tbsp lime juice

1 Chop the fruit and mix together in a bowl.
2 Combine the honey and lime juice and stir this into the mixed fruit.
3 Place in the fridge to cool until ready to serve in your lunchbox.

Simple Apple Crumble

Crumble is one of the simplest desserts to make and is delicious eaten cold. These simple little crumbles are so comforting in the middle of the day.

MAKES 4 PORTIONS

2 tbsp of butter or coconut oil
2 eating apples
½ tsp of cinnamon
2 tbsp honey
50g oats

1 Preheat the oven to 200°C/Fan 180°C/Gas 6.
2 Heat the butter or coconut oil in a saucepan. Slice the apples up into slithers (I find an apple wedger works well here) and add the apples to the pan. Cook over a low heat for a few minutes, stirring. Add in the cinnamon and honey. Place the lid on the saucepan and cook gently for up to 10 minutes – just until the apple slices are cooked through.
3 Place the apple slices in 4 small ramekins, leaving the cooking juices in the pan.
4 Stir the oats into the leftover juices, until the juices are all soaked up and the oats coated.
5 Add the oats to the ramekins and push down over the sliced apples with the back of a spoon.
6 Bake the crumbles for 15 minutes in the oven.
7 Remove and leave to cool before serving in your lunchbox.

6 Souper Douper

Why Soups for Lunch?

Soups are not just suitable for lunches, they're ideal. Yet they often get forgotten about when it comes to lunchboxes, perhaps because of preconceived ideas of what a lunchbox should contain. Soups vary hugely but they can make a whole nutritionally balanced meal in terms of both macronutrients (carbohydrates, proteins and fats) and micronutrients (vitamins and minerals) in their own right. You might, however, choose to serve your soup with accompaniments, such as bread or croutons or alongside other lunchbox foods.

The reasons that soups are such an ideal lunchbox food is that they are:

Timesavers

Soups save time because they bubble away on the kitchen stove or even in your pressure cooker, if you are lucky enough to have one, while you get on with something else. Once the basic components have been added in the right order the soup itself can just simmer gently as those delicious flavours develop.

Easy to Make

There's a simple formula to follow for virtually every soup. It's a building process, adding layers of flavour and texture as you go. This step-by-step process is outlined on the next page.

An Opportunity to Eat More Vegetables

Soups provide a great opportunity to consume more vegetables. While some people have an aversion to certain vegetables whole or uncooked, they might not even notice them once cooked down in a soup. Often, they may actually like the flavour of the vegetable once it's part of a soup. Perfect examples of this include the vast number of people who don't like eating tomatoes or mushrooms but love tomato soup or mushroom soup. Soups allow for the addition of lots of vegetables both for flavour and texture.

Help to Broaden Palates

It is because soups can contain a variety of previously unloved vegetables and ingredients that there is the opportunity to stretch the breadth of flavours you or your child are willing to try. A soup can introduce your taste buds to different regions or countries of the world, for example with a Thai soup or curried soup.

Help Save Vegetables From Waste

Do you often find there are vegetables left in your fridge that you simply don't know how to use up? They'll be great in your next soup. So many of us throw vegetables away simply because we can't think of a way to eat them. Whether it's a shallot, sticks of celery, a carrot or perhaps even something more obscure. You can simply chop it up and add it at the appropriate time to the soup – it will provide flavour and texture and clear out your cupboards/fridge. It's a win-win.

Let's talk about building that soup, layer upon layer. It really is as simple as follows:

Step One – Aromatics

One of my fondest childhood memories is the smell of carrots and leeks sautéing gently in the pan. A soup that we used to eat regularly was called Potage Bonne Femme although we never knew it by that fancy name. To us it was just leek and potato soup. That smell can transport me back to the 1980s in a jiff. I didn't quite know it at the time but watching Mum make that soup was teaching me the first lesson in soup-making. That is to choose your favourite aromatics and sauté them gently. By aromatics I mean leeks, onions, shallots, carrots, celery, ginger or garlic. Choose any combination of these as your starting point. The choice of oil is up to you, but personally I love the smell and taste of vegetables sautéed in butter. I regularly use olive oil in soups these days too.

If you are wondering which oil or fat to cook with then look no further. Always choose real fats to cook in rather than manufactured and refined polyunsaturated oils such as sunflower or vegetable oil. Saturated fats, thanks to their molecular structure, are heat stable. You can identify saturated fat readily because it stays solid at room temperature. Due to its stability, saturated fat is not as subject to oxidation as the less stable polyunsaturated oils. Saturated fats are not chemically altered by cooking and so are suitable for high- and low-heat cooking. These fats include butter, ghee and coconut oil.

Olive and avocado oils should, in theory, be unstable when heated as they are monounsaturated, yet they both contain polyphenols and tocopherols which act to protect the oils from oxidation. Another reason they are stable is because they're made up of mostly monounsaturated fat. That means they're more stable in heat than fats with high amounts of polyunsaturated fats which have more double bonds. Thanks to these two properties, olive and avocado oils can both be used at higher heats than you might have thought. These two oils, olive and avocado, are recommended for cooking the base of your soup or indeed any cooked meal in the Hot Meals chapter (p.96).

Step Two – Choose Your Liquid/Stock
While many of us favour the convenience of stock cubes, pots and gels these days – and these certainly do provide flavour – be sure to check the ingredients for allergens and ingredients that you don't recognise. There are some better stock cubes and pots on the market, but you have to choose discerningly.

It is also possible to use other liquids in addition to or in place of stock cubes and pots. The water left over from boiling or steaming vegetables, bone broth, home-made stock, soy sauce, tamari and just plain water are all options.

Additionally, you may choose to use a pre-prepared paste such as Thai curry paste, Indian curry paste, harissa paste, chipotle paste, tomato paste, miso or sun-dried tomato paste alongside your stock and/or water for a particular taste.

Step Three – Add Your Feature Ingredient
This is most likely to be the ingredient after which your soup is named. This ingredient could be meat-based such as chorizo, ham, bacon, beef, lamb, chicken; fish-based such as haddock or prawns; or it could be vegetable-based such as sweet potato, butternut squash, celeriac, cauliflower, mushroom, pea or sweetcorn. You could even combine both meat or fish- and vegetable-feature ingredients.

Step Four – Add in Your Texture Providers
Texture can be provided by a range of ingredients, from noodles, pasta, rice and potatoes to pulses, such as lentils, split peas and chickpeas. Pulses provide fibre, protein, calcium, potassium, folate, zinc, iron and magnesium. Noodles, pasta, rice and potatoes provide carbohydrates, which we burn for energy, and if reheated produce something called

resistant starch, which we are just starting to understand the role of in improving digestive health. Using precooked pasta, rice and potatoes in soups therefore provides health advantages. Alongside vegetables these additions make for a delicious and nutritious meal.

Step Five – Finesse the Flavour

This step is about bringing the flavour of the soup together. It is best to taste test at this point to see what else needs to be added. It's even better if you can get the opinion of others too. Here is an idea of which herbs and spices work best with which vegetables:

Mushrooms: garlic, sage
Peas: marjoram, mint
Potatoes: chives, cumin, dill, fennel, garlic, mace, rosemary, tarragon
Squashes/sweet potatoes: cardamom, coriander, cumin, ginger, nutmeg
Tomatoes: allspice, basil, cloves, cumin, fennel, marjoram, oregano

At this stage, you might also choose to add other flavour providers, such as citrus juice, vinegar, cheese, salt and pepper.

Step Six – To Blend or Not to Blend?

In my experience, soups such as tomato and vegetable lend themselves to being blended, while those with pasta, rice or noodles do not. It's totally up to you and those eating the soup to decide. Just remember that for most blenders the soup will need to be cooled before you blend it. Also, remember not to overfill the blender with soup. Soup disasters are most likely to happen when the soup is too hot or if you have overfilled the blender.

Step Seven – Choose What to Serve with the Soup

A young child faced with a large container of soup is often overwhelmed. However, serving some chunks of absorbent bread – sourdough is ideal for this purpose – alongside can certainly help. Most adults enjoy bread with soup too. If the soup contains noodles or rice, they too will absorb more of the liquid over time, so if you are serving the soup in a flask and it's not going to be eaten until lunchtime there may be a significant reduction in liquid. For many this is a good thing because it makes the whole dish easier to eat.

Recipes

The soup recipes in this chapter are hugely varied, so there's bound to be something to suit your taste buds. They're all designed to contribute vegetables to the lunchbox. If you are making hot soups to take to work or school you'll need a flask, so do check out the Using Insulated Flasks Effectively section in the Hot Meals chapter on p.96.

Sourdough Croutons

These little crunchy croutons make the perfect addition to hot soups and stews. I recommend transporting them to school or work in a separate container from the soup so they don't go soggy. Then add them to the top of the flask of soup when it's time for lunch.

50g sourdough bread, cut into 2cm cubes
1 tsp olive oil
(you can also use garlic, chilli or herb-infused oils for a little added flavour)

1   Preheat the oven to 200°C/Fan 180°C/Gas 6.
2   Spread the bread cubes out on to a baking tray and drizzle over a teaspoon of olive oil.
3   Bake in the oven for 10 minutes until golden and crispy.

Basic Vegetable Soup

If you are not sure where to start, here is a basic recipe that can be adapted to your taste preferences. With practice and familiarity, you'll become a super-confident soup-maker using this process as your base.

SERVES 4–6

2 tbsp olive oil
1 onion, diced
1 garlic clove, peeled and crushed
1 celery stick, sliced
550g fresh vegetables, peeled and diced
1 medium potato, peeled and diced
1 stock cube
Salt and pepper

1   Heat the oil in a large saucepan.
2   Fry the onion, garlic and celery until soft but not brown.
3   Add the vegetables and cook until mildly soft.
4   Add the diced potato.
5   Add the stock cube and 900ml of water.
6   Simmer for 15–20 minutes. Check the vegetables are all cooked.
7   Leave the soup to cool, before whizzing it up in a food processor until smooth, or just leave as is.
8   Season to taste.
9   Reheat before placing the soup in warmed flasks for lunch (see Using Insulated Flasks Effectively on p.96 for how to warm your flask).

Sweetcorn Chowder

This soup is simply bursting with flavour. This recipe harnesses corn's natural sweetness to become an integral part of this delicious and nutritious creamy soup.

SERVES 4–6

1 tbsp olive oil
2 onions, chopped
2 carrots, chopped
2 celery sticks, chopped
900ml vegetable stock
500g frozen sweetcorn
2 tbsp creamed coconut or 3 tbsp full-fat milk

1   Heat the olive oil in a large saucepan.
2   Add the chopped onions. Stir and continue to cook until they start to become transparent.
3   Add the carrots and celery and stir for a couple of minutes.
4   Add the stock and bring to the boil.
5   When the vegetables are almost cooked, add the sweetcorn and continue to cook for a further 10 minutes.
6   Turn off the heat and stir in the creamed coconut or milk.
7   Leave the soup to cool before popping it into a food processor. Leave the soup fairly chunky so that it retains some texture.
8   Reheat before placing the soup in warmed flasks for lunch.

Chocolate Bean Chilli Soup

Thanks to Jo Keyes from Time to Nourish for this addition to the book. Jo is a very talented naturopathic chef who has three children of her own. She has created this hearty soup which is a plant-based twist on the traditional Mexican dish Pozole Rojo. Bursting with flavour and packed full of protein-rich beans and colourful veg, this dish will satisfy anyone needing a nutritious on-the-go meal.

SERVES 4–6

For the chocolate chilli paste
5 ancho dried chillies
500ml warm water
2 tbsp cacao powder
40g sun-dried tomatoes in olive oil, drained
1 medjool date, pitted
5 small garlic cloves, peeled and halved
100g tinned chopped tomatoes

For the chilli
2 tbsp olive oil
1 large onion, diced
1 red pepper, deseeded and diced
1 courgette, diced
1 tbsp tamari
1 tbsp oregano
2 tsp cumin
¼ tsp salt
200g tinned sweetcorn, drained
400g tinned black beans, drained and rinsed
500ml hot water
2 tsp vegetable bouillon powder (vegetable stock powder)
Juice of ½ lime

1   Remove the stalks and deseed the dried chillies, then soak them in the warm water for 20 minutes.
2   Add the soaked chillies and soaking water to a high-powered blender along with the cacao powder, sun-dried tomatoes, date,

garlic cloves and tinned tomatoes, then blend until smooth.

3   Heat the oil in a large saucepan then add the onion and pepper and sauté for 2 minutes.

4   Add the courgette and sauté for a further 2 minutes.

5   Mix the tamari, oregano, cumin and salt in a small bowl, then add this to the vegetables and stir to combine and cook for 2 more minutes.

6   Add the sweetcorn, black beans and chocolate chilli paste and stir to combine.

7   Mix 500ml of hot water (or less if you prefer a thicker chilli) with bouillon powder until dissolved and then add the liquid to the pot, stirring to combine.

8   Bring to the boil and simmer, uncovered, for 15 minutes, stirring occasionally.

9   Add the lime juice, then taste to check the seasoning and adjust to your liking.

10   Serve with your chosen toppings and a side of sour dough or add some brown basmati rice.

Topping ideas: Why not garnish with some fresh coriander, radish, avocado, spring onion, white or green cabbage?

Mushroom Soup

Mushrooms – love them or hate them? There are few foods that seem to create such extreme reactions as mushrooms. If you are a mushroom lover then you'll enjoy this soup, which combines the classic flavours of garlic and mushroom. Even if you are not a fan of mushrooms – perhaps because of their texture – then this soup may be perfect for you. This is all about that deep umami flavour.

SERVES 2–4

40g salted butter
1 large onion, chopped
2 garlic cloves, crushed
300g large flat mushrooms, chopped
1 tbsp soy sauce or tamari (gluten-free)
330ml milk (dairy-free or lactose-free optional)
2 tbsp chopped parsley

1   Melt the butter in a large saucepan over a medium heat. Sauté the onions until soft.
2   Add the garlic and mushrooms and stir until the mushrooms start to release their own liquid.
3   Add the soy sauce or tamari and 330ml of water.
4   Bring to the boil then simmer, uncovered, for 20 minutes.
5   Stir in the milk and parsley then leave to cool. Use a food processor to process but not on full speed – you still want some texture left in this soup.
6   Reheat before placing the soup in warmed flasks for lunch.

Carrot and Leek Soup

During the winter months when there is less local, seasonal produce available, two vegetables that are usually available are carrots and leeks. Together they make a delicious soup. This is an ideal winter warmer!

SERVES 4–6

4 large carrots, peeled and thickly sliced
2 tbsp olive oil
2 tbsp butter
4 leeks, sliced in half lengthways, then cut into half discs
4 tsp vegetable bouillon powder (vegetable stock powder)
1 litre hot water
50ml milk (optional)

1   Preheat the oven to 200°C/Fan 180°C/Gas 6.
2   Lay the carrot slices on a baking sheet. Drizzle over the olive oil. Roast the carrots for 30–35 minutes, until they are soft. Turn once while they are roasting.
3   Meanwhile, melt the butter, add the leeks and allow these to cook slowly in a large lidded saucepan. Stir until they are soft and starting to caramelise slightly. This should take about 10 minutes.
4   Mix the vegetable bouillon with the hot water.
5   Once the carrots are roasted and the leeks softened put the bouillon and carrots into the pan with the leeks.
6   Simmer for 10–15 minutes then leave to cool before processing everything in a food processor. You can add milk at this stage if you want a creamier soup.
7   Warm the soup through again and pour into warmed flasks.

Chicken Noodle Soup

A childhood classic! Though the version I had as a child was from a packet and full of salt. This version is much simpler and makes for a really filling lunchbox classic made from real-food ingredients.

SERVES 4–6

1 tbsp olive oil
1 onion, chopped
1 garlic clove, finely chopped or crushed
2 skinless, boneless free-range chicken breasts, sliced
3 carrots, diced
575ml vegetable stock or 1 stock cube and 575ml water
About 125g rice noodles (uncooked weight)

1   In a medium saucepan, heat the olive oil then sauté the onion for 2 minutes. Add the garlic and stir.
2   Next add the chicken breast and cook for about 4 minutes. Then add the carrots and the stock together. Cover and simmer for about 15 minutes.
3   Meanwhile, bring another saucepan to the boil. Add the rice noodles and cook for 5 minutes (or according to the packet instructions), until soft and ready to eat. Drain, rinse (to get rid of the excess starch) then add the noodles to the chicken and carrot soup pan.
4   You might like to remove and shred the chicken further at this point then add it back to the soup.
5   Pack the soup into warmed flasks for lunch.

Note: rice noodles packed in soup in this way will continue to absorb some of the liquid. This makes for less liquid by lunchtime but this by no means detracts from the taste or enjoyment of the dish.

Thai Sweet Potato and Lentil Soup

Subtle but slightly sweet Thai flavours combine with the creamy lentils to make for a tasty and filling soup.

SERVES 4–6

2 tbsp olive oil
1 onion, chopped
1–2 tbsp red Thai curry paste
3cm piece of root ginger, grated
750g sweet potato, peeled and diced
160g split red lentils, rinsed
1 litre vegetable stock or stock cubes and water
1 tbsp lime juice
2 tsp coconut sugar
200g coconut milk
Salt and pepper

1   Heat the olive oil in a medium-sized saucepan over a medium heat then add the onion and saute, stirring regularly.
2   When the onion becomes soft, add the curry paste and ginger. Heat through for another few minutes then add the sweet potato cubes and the red lentils with the stock, lime juice and sugar. Season to taste.
3   Bring to the boil and then simmer for 20 minutes.
4   Add the coconut milk and stir. Once cool, use a stick blender or food processor to blend to a smoother consistency. Warm through then place in a warmed flask.

Cauliflower and Bacon Soup

The sweet and salty flavours from the cauliflower and bacon really complement each other in this soup recipe. Cooking and blending the cauliflower results in a satisfyingly creamy soup.

SERVES 4–6

1 tbsp olive oil
1 onion, roughly chopped
3 rashers of unsmoked back bacon, thinly sliced
1 garlic clove, chopped
1 large cauliflower, chopped into large florets
1 tbsp tamari/soy sauce

1   Heat the oil in a saucepan then add the onion and bacon. Stir regularly while they cook until the onion becomes translucent. Then add the garlic, cauliflower, tamari or soy sauce and 800ml of water.
2   Put a lid on the saucepan and bring the liquid to the boil then reduce the heat and simmer for about 10–15 minutes or until the cauliflower is just soft. Don't overcook this as the cauliflower will become mushy and flavourless.
3   Leave to cool then use a food processor to blend everything to a creamy consistency. Heat up in portion sizes and pour into warmed flasks.

Top tip: Buy frozen chopped garlic and keep it in the freezer until you need it. This is quicker, often fresher and results in cleaner (and less garlicky) hands.

Pea and Broccoli Soup

Not everyone loves their greens, but the sweet, fresh flavour
in this soup might persuade those doubters otherwise.
The sweet-tasting peas and chickpeas give a satisfying,
wholesome texture to the soup, too.

SERVES 4

1 tbsp butter
1 tbsp olive oil
1 onion, roughly chopped
½ a large head of broccoli, chopped into florets
750ml vegetable stock
A few sprigs of thyme
60g garden peas
½ x 400g tin of chickpeas, drained
Salt and pepper

1   Melt the butter and oil in a large pan and gently fry the onion
    until soft.
2   Add the broccoli, followed by the stock and thyme.
3   Bring to the boil then simmer until the broccoli is tender.
4   Remove the thyme from the pot.
5   Add the peas and chickpeas and stir until the peas are
    defrosted. Once cool, process everything in a food processor
    until smooth.
6   Bring back up to temperature, season to taste and pour into
    warmed flasks.

Pea and Mint Soup

A British staple, this dish is loved by many. Made with a classic combination of flavours – pea and mint – this bright green soup is immensely appealing in both appearance and flavour.

SERVES 2–4

1 tbsp butter or olive oil
1 large onion, chopped
1 garlic clove, chopped
400g frozen peas
500ml vegetable stock
2 tbsp chopped mint
2 tbsp cream cheese
Salt and pepper

1 Heat the oil or butter in a large saucepan.
2 Add the onion and garlic and cook until the onion is transparent.
3 Add the peas and stir.
4 Add the stock. Bring it up to the boil.
5 Turn off the heat, add in the mint and the cream cheese and leave to cool a little, then process in a food processor to the desired consistency.
6 Check the seasoning then reheat and pour into warmed flasks.

Simple Tomato Soup

As tomato soup seems to be a favourite for many, especially
those new to the concept of transporting soup for lunch,
I am including this extremely simple but effective recipe for
home-made tomato soup. The inclusion of bread thickens it and
makes this a suitably filling lunchtime meal.

SERVES 2–4

4 tbsp olive oil
1 x 400g carton of passata
2 garlic cloves
1 tsp mixed dried herbs
2 slices of medium-thickness wholemeal bread (gluten-free optional)
1–1½ tbsp honey
Pinch of salt

1   Heat the olive oil in a medium-sized saucepan.
2   Add the passata and garlic with the mixed herbs and 250ml of
     water.
3   Bring this to the boil then reduce and simmer until the soup
     gets thicker.
4   Rip the bread into chunks and add this along with another
     250ml of water.
5   Add the honey and a pinch of salt.
6   Bring to the boil again, then cover the saucepan and turn the
     heat off.
7   Pour into warmed flasks.

Roasted Sweet Potato, Pepper and Coconut Soup

This soup is a full-on flavour explosion – it brings together the sweetness of roasted sweet potato and red pepper and coconut cream into a taste extravaganza of a soup.

SERVES 2

1 large sweet potato, peeled and chopped into roughly 2cm cubes
1 red pepper, chopped into thick strips
1 red onion, cut into quarters
2 garlic cloves, whole but peeled
1 tsp sweet smoked paprika, plus extra for serving
1 tsp salt
2 tbsp olive oil
160ml coconut cream, plus extra for serving
300ml vegetable stock
(if using stock cubes, use less salt earlier in the recipe)

1   Preheat the oven to 200°C/Fan 180°C/Gas 6.
2   Toss all the vegetables and the garlic in a bowl with the paprika, salt and oil.
3   Place everything on a baking tray and roast until soft – this should take about 25 minutes.
4   Leave to cool then put everything into a food processor along with the coconut cream and stock. Process until no chunky bits are left.
5   Reheat in a saucepan before placing into warm flasks. Add a swirl of coconut cream and a sprinkling of sweet smoked paprika to the top of the soup if desired.

Cauliflower Cheese Soup

Another classic flavour pairing: cauliflower and cheese. This soup recreates a childhood favourite dish but in a soup.

SERVES 4–6

1 tbsp butter
1 onion, chopped
¼ tsp mustard powder
1 large cauliflower (about 900g), broken into small florets
600ml organic milk
150ml vegetable stock
2 tsp olive oil
100g mature Cheddar cheese, grated
Salt and pepper

1   Melt the butter in a large saucepan. Add the onion and cook over a medium heat for 3 minutes, stirring frequently.
2   Sprinkle over the mustard and stir it in.
3   Add the cauliflower to the saucepan together with the milk and stock. Bring to the boil, then reduce the heat. Cover and simmer for 10 minutes or until the cauliflower is tender.
4   Leave to cool then process in a food processor. Season with salt and pepper to taste, then reheat until just bubbling.
5   Add the grated cheese and stir until melted. Pour into warmed flasks.

Butternut Squash and Feta Soup

Sweet and buttery butternut squash works well alongside creamy, soft feta cheese in this simple soup.

1 tbsp olive oil
2 small red onions, sliced
300g butternut squash, peeled and deseeded then chopped into roughly 2cm cubes
1 clove of garlic, crushed
500ml vegetable stock
100g feta

1   Heat the olive oil in a large saucepan.
2   Sauté the red onion until soft and transparent then add the squash and garlic. Cover with the stock then bring to the boil, reduce the heat and simmer for 15 minutes.
3   Leave to cool a little then blend in a food processor before pouring the soup back into the pan to heat through. Pour into warmed flasks with crumbled feta cheese over the top.

Potage Bonne Femme

Earlier in this chapter I mentioned memories of my mum cooking up a classic French soup made from a base of sautéed leeks and carrots. It seems only fitting that I should end this chapter with the recipe I remember most fondly from my own childhood.

SERVES 6

30g butter
3 medium carrots, diced (roughly)
2 large leeks, finely sliced
450g potatoes, peeled and diced into 3cm cubes
Up to 1 tsp unrefined sugar, to season
2 tbsp cream
Salt and pepper

1   Heat the butter in a large pan, add the carrots and leeks and stir regularly.
2   Once the leeks are softening, add the potatoes, 1.2 litres of water and some salt, pepper and a little sugar.
3   Leave uncovered to simmer for 20–25 minutes, until the potatoes are soft.
4   Remove the pan from the heat and leave to cool slightly, then blend in a food processor until the soup is perfectly smooth.
5   Check the seasoning then pour in the cream, stir and pour into warmed flasks.

7 Hot Meals

The Value of Insulated Flasks

An insulated food or drink flask opens up a world of opportunities when it comes to portable lunches. It's a great way of serving leftovers for one thing. I know I am not alone in thinking that cooked food often tastes even more delicious the day after it was first prepared.

Hot food at lunch is also rather comforting. It may be cold, grey and miserable outside, but you have the warmth and comfort of a home cooked meal inside your flask. It doesn't have to be a home-cooked meal though. There's nothing stopping you packing shop-bought meals, soups, stews and curries. These can be heated up at home and transported to work, saving you time, energy and money at lunchtime rather than trying to find something to buy to eat in the limited time you have available. There are many options, both home-cooked or shop-bought.

Ensuring that you have each of the six components of a balanced lunch (see p.8) becomes far easier when you include a hot meal in a flask as part of the overall meal. Inevitably, a hot meal, especially those made of leftovers, contains more than one of the six food groups and often three or four.

Using Insulated Flasks Effectively

Those new to using insulated flasks for children or themselves may be unsure how to get the most out of them. There are some simple steps to follow to ensure your food stays warm until lunchtime and tastes great.

Hand Wash:

Hand washing your flasks is recommended. Some are dishwasher-proof, but even so, dishwashing can cause the flask to degrade sooner. Wash with warm soapy water and rinse clean of any residual detergent. Ensure you wash the inside thoroughly but also the lid, and remove the seal to clean that too if possible.

Pre-warm:

Whenever possible, warm the flask before packing it with your hot food. This way the food will keep warmer for longer. Pour freshly boiled water into the flask and close the lid. Allow that to sit in there for up to ten minutes while you prepare your lunch. Remove the lid, pour out the water and pack in your hot food. By putting your food into a warm flask, the food will stay warm and won't start to cool down straight away.

Do Not Overfill:
There are two reasons not to overfill your flask. Hot food is obviously a burning/scalding hazard. Secondly, if any food is left on or near the seal or lid, it can prevent the lid from sealing properly and that means the food could spill and will also cool down far more quickly.

Size:
- For younger children, a food flask that holds about 300ml is suitable.
- For older children and adults, flasks with a 450–500ml capacity are more suitable.

Choosing a Hot Meal for Lunch

Soup
Soup as a lunchtime food is covered in the previous chapter (p.75), in which you will find plenty of soup preparation tips and techniques as well as suitable lunchtime soup recipes. Suffice to say, there are also plenty of fresh soup brands on the market for all sorts of budgets, as well as healthier brands available in tins.

Always check the ingredients labels for ingredients you do not recognise. Watch out for added sugars as some brands add sugar to please the modern palate (some tomato soups can have 3½ teaspoons of sugar per half a can, for example) and be particularly aware of added salt. Some ready-made soups contain 2.5–3g of salt per portion.

According to MHS guidelines, we should be eating no more than 6g of salt, which equates to 2.4g of sodium per day. Those numbers need to be reduced according to the age of your children as follows:

	Adult	Child 7–10yrs	Child 4–6yrs	Child 1–3yrs
Salt	6g	5g	3g	2g
Sodium	2.4g	2g	1.2g	0.8g

Pulse-based Dishes

A pulse-based meal at lunchtime can add some plant-based protein to your diet, especially important if you do not consume meat. Pulses include peas, beans and lentils. In fact, even the word 'pulse' is derived from the Latin words *puls* or *pultis* meaning 'thick soup'. Pulses provide about 10 per cent of the total dietary protein consumed in the world and have about twice the protein content of most cereal grains. They offer the nutritional advantage of not only being high in protein but also fibre, as well as being simple to prepare and lower in cost. Bean, pea and lentil dishes that warm you up and power you through even the toughest afternoon of school or work could include black bean chilli, baked beans or chickpea curry.

Pasta Lunch

Pasta-based lunches are carbohydrate-rich and comforting on chilly days. The way you cook your pasta and the type of pasta you choose affects the rate at which energy is released from pasta dishes. Make these meals healthier and ensure they provide you with longer-lasting energy by using wholegrain spelt pasta, brown rice pasta, pulse-based pastas (those made from chickpea or lentil), or even vegetable pastas such as courgette spaghetti.

Try not to overcook your pasta. It should be al dente (slightly firm and chewy); that way it can be considered a slower-release carbohydrate. The Italian phrase '*al dente*' in fact means 'firm to the bite'.

Sauces are key to ensuring the pasta stays deliciously moist until lunchtime. Ensure the pasta is evenly coated in sauce whatever type and whatever sauce you are using. If you want cheese on top of the pasta you are better off transporting this separately and scattering over the contents of the flask just before you eat, otherwise it can melt into a mass, making the dish far less appealing come lunchtime.

Chilli Lunch

Chillies are far more diverse than just our classic take on chilli-con-carne. You can vary the protein source from chicken, turkey or venison mince through to various types of beans and lentils, and you can add vegetables galore to bulk up the chilli while also boosting its nutritional value. A wholesome chilli could be the centre-piece of a delicious and nutritious lunch, but you could also serve accompaniments, such as guacamole, corn tortillas, salsa, sour cream or yogurt, cheese or lettuce to make the whole lunchtime experience a little more authentic.

Curries

Like chillies, curries can be varied, and they really don't have to be spicy hot. Using aromatic spices rather than chilli in your curry can create the subtlest of curried flavours.

The protein source can vary from meat, fish and even eggs through to beans, lentils and chickpeas. Although there are many different types of curry, they tend to have basic ingredients in common: onion, ginger, garlic, spices and a liquid base. If you fancy trying some curries in lunches here is a simple step-by-step process:

STEP 1: Heat 1 tbsp of oil (ghee, coconut oil or avocado oil) in a pan.

STEP 2: Add 1 chopped onion and cook until transparent.

STEP 3: Add 1-2 tsp of grated ginger and 2 cloves of minced garlic.

STEP 4: Add salt and your choice of spices (ground cumin, turmeric, coriander, cinnamon, curry power, and even some chilli powder and or cayenne pepper if you want some heat).

STEP 5: Add meat and/or vegetables and pulses, as well as some liquid (coconut milk, tomatoes – tinned, canned or from a carton – and stock).

STEP 6: Add something to thicken the curry (tomato purée, ground almonds, yogurt, coconut cream).

STEP 7: Simmer until the vegetables and/or meat are cooked through.

STEP 8: Pop the curry into your warmed flasks and enjoy for lunch or leave it to cool and enjoy for multiple lunches over the next few days.

Protein in Hot Lunches

One of the many advantages of taking hot cooked food to work or school is that it provides an opportunity for good-quality proteins in sufficient amounts. A more typical lunch made up of mostly bread and crisps provides an abundance of refined carbohydrates and often too little protein and, as we know, this can lead to energy dips. So, providing a hot cooked lunch with sufficient protein will do wonders for consistent afternoon energy levels.

For children, you can work out their ideal protein intake by multiplying their weight in pounds by 0.5, or simply take their weight in pounds and divide by 2. For instance, a 70-pound child should have about 35 grams of protein every day. If you only know your weight in kilograms, you need about 1 gram of protein each day for every kilogram you weigh.

For young adults and adults the following applies:

MALES	Recommended daily protein intake (for average age and weight)	Specific intake recommended per kg of body weight
14–18 years	65g	0.99g/kg
19–70 years	64g	0.84/kg
70 and above	81g	1.07g/kg

FEMALES	Recommended daily protein intake (for average age and weight)	Specific intake recommended per kg of body weight
14–18 years	45g	0.77g/kg
19–70 years	46g	0.75/kg
70 and above	57g	1.07g/kg
Pregnant	60g	1.00g/kg
Lactating	67g	1.10g/kg

When you buy products from the shop you can look at the food label to find out how much protein in grams is in a serving. If you are unsure how much protein is in common foods, then this should help:

Food	How much you need to get 20g of protein
Yogurt (natural)	125g (small) pot
Eggs	2 medium
Salmon	100g (1 small piece)
Cod	35g (very small piece)
Sardines	100g (1 sardine)
Chicken	75g (small breast)
Tinned tuna	85g (small tin)
Tofu	275g (¾ pack)
Brown rice	400g (cooked weight)
Lentils	85g (cooked weight)
Quinoa	100g (dry weight)
Almonds	115g
Cashew nuts	115g
Pumpkin seeds	75g
Sunflower seeds	185g
Pulses (peas, chickpeas, lentils and beans)	100g

Recipes

The following recipes are designed to provide a range of substantial hot meals that are not only delicious and nutritious but can be enjoyed at work or school.

Moroccan Lamb

This dish has the flavours of Morocco. Mince-based dishes are easy and cost-effective on the whole and this dish is no different. In this case, the lamb combines with the sweet flavours of onion, sweet potato and tomato. The dish should be served in a flask but ideally with some form of flatbread for dipping. Some might also like a little natural yogurt too.

SERVES 4–6

1 tsp olive oil
2 onions, chopped
500g minced lamb
1 tbsp harissa paste
1 x 400g tin of chickpeas, drained and rinsed
1 x 400g tin of chopped tomatoes
500g sweet potatoes, peeled and cubed into roughly 2cm pieces
2 courgettes, thickly sliced

1   Heat the oil in a large saucepan and then add the onions and fry these gently until they become transparent.
2   Add the mince and harissa paste and cook for a further 10 minutes.
3   Add the chickpeas, tomatoes and sweet potatoes and simmer for 20 minutes.
4   Add the courgettes and simmer for a further 10 minutes.
5   Divide into warmed flasks.

Serving suggestion: a small pot of yogurt and a flatbread.

Black Bean Chilli

Black beans are a deliciously filling vegetable protein and they lend themselves to Mexican-style dishes really well. This chilli is mild enough for most palates, but for those particularly sensitive to heat go easy on the chipotle.

SERVES 2–4

1 tbsp olive oil
1 onion, diced
1 garlic clove, crushed
1 tsp chipotle paste
2 carrots, grated
1 courgette, grated
400g passata
¼ tsp ground cinnamon
¼ tsp ground coriander
½ tsp salt
2 tbsp tomato purée
1 x 400g tin of black beans, drained and rinsed

1 Heat the oil in a large pan over a medium heat.
2 Sauté the onion until transparent.
3 Add the garlic and chipotle paste and stir for a minute.
4 Now add the carrots and courgette and stir for 2 minutes.
5 Add the passata, spices, salt and tomato purée and cook for 10 minutes, stirring regularly.
6 Add the black beans and stir, then pop a lid on and turn the heat off to allow the beans to warm through.
7 Pop into warmed flasks.

Serving suggestion: a small pot of yogurt, grated cheese and some sliced avocado.

Chickpea and Vegetable Curry

Chickpeas are another filling vegetarian protein. They are extremely versatile and commonly used in Asian and Middle Eastern cuisine. This curry recipe is very simple with few ingredients and even fewer steps. You can certainly jazz it up a bit. I like to add more vegetables, but I appreciate not everyone loves to see lots of green in their curry.

SERVES 2–4

1 tbsp olive oil
1 onion, diced
1 garlic clove, crushed
1 heaped tsp medium curry powder
½ a courgette, diced to the same sized pieces as the onion (optional)
1 x 400g tin of chickpeas, drained and rinsed
½ x 400g tin of chopped tomatoes
½ tsp salt or half a vegetable stock cube
100g fresh spinach, rinsed and dried

1 Heat the oil in a medium-sized saucepan.
2 Sauté the onion for 5 minutes.
3 After 5 minutes add the garlic and the curry powder. Stir.
4 Stir in the courgette, chickpeas and tomatoes with 125ml of water, the salt or ½ a vegetable stock cube, and the spinach.
5 Bring to the boil (pushing the spinach into the saucepan as you go until it has wilted) then reduce the heat and simmer for 20 minutes, until the sauce is significantly reduced. Place in warmed flasks.

Minced Beef and Sweet Potato Curry

If you like the mild and fruity taste of bolognese then you will surely enjoy this mild minced beef and sweet potato curry too.

SERVES 4–6

1 tbsp olive oil
1 onion, chopped
1 garlic clove, minced
1¼ tsp grated ginger
400g minced beef
1 medium sweet potato (about 200g), chopped into 1cm cubes
1 medium courgette (about 170g), chopped into 2cm cubes
1 tsp sea salt
15g medium curry powder
1 x 400g tin of tomatoes
1 tbsp tomato paste

1   Heat the oil in a large saucepan over a medium heat.
2   Sauté the onion until transparent. Add the garlic and ginger and stir to combine.
3   Add the beef and stir until browned.
4   Add the sweet potato, courgette, salt, curry powder, tinned tomatoes and tomato paste and bring to the boil with the lid on. Then leave to simmer with the lid on for 20 minutes or until the sweet potato is cooked.
5   Place in warmed flasks.

Chicken Curry

Chicken curry is probably most people's introduction to the world of curry. This is a very mild and gentle curry fit for lunches at work or school.

2 tbsp olive oil
2 small onions, diced
1 celery stick, diced
1 garlic clove, thinly sliced
2 tbsp mild curry paste
1 stock cube
2 medium sweet potatoes, peeled and cubed
400g can of coconut milk
2 chicken breasts, cubed
100g frozen peas

1   Heat the olive oil in a medium pan over a medium heat.
2   Sauté the onions, celery and garlic until soft.
3   Stir in the curry paste.
4   Add the stock cube, sweet potato cubes and coconut milk. Bring to a simmer and simmer for 15 minutes.
5   Add the chicken and simmer for a further 15 minutes.
6   Add the peas, stir, then cover with a lid and switch off the heat.
7   Place in warmed flasks.

Beef and Vegetable Burgers

The grated vegetables in these burgers not only add to their nutritional value and make the ingredients go a little further – they also add incredible flavour and texture.

MAKES 4 BURGERS

½ medium carrot
½ medium courgette
½ garlic clove
20g flavoursome cheese such as pecorino, finely grated
Handful of fresh parsley, finely chopped
250g minced beef
Black pepper

1   Finely grate the carrot, courgette and garlic, squeezing as much water out of them as possible, ideally through a piece of muslin.
2   Preheat the grill to medium.
3   Combine the grated vegetables, cheese, parsley and mince with a good twist of black pepper.
4   Mould into 4 equal-sized beef burgers.
5   Grill under a medium heat, until cooked through. Pop into warmed flasks with some roasted sweet potato wedges.

Vegetable Bolognese

Technically speaking a bolognese is a tomato sauce to which meat is added, so strictly speaking this is not a bolognese sauce, but it can be used in the same way. That is to say it can be enjoyed alongside pasta and its texture actually comes from vegetables rather than meat. More vegetables is always a good thing!

SERVES 2–4

1 aubergine, roughly chopped
1 courgette, roughly chopped
1 celery stick, roughly chopped
2 medium carrots, roughly chopped
1 onion, roughly chopped
2 tbsp olive oil
4 tomatoes, quartered
1 vegetable stock cube
400ml passata
200–400g cooked pasta (roughly 100g cooked pasta per serving)
Salt and pepper (optional)

1   Whizz all the chopped vegetables, except the tomatoes, in a food processor to form a rough pulp.
2   Place the olive oil in a thick-based frying pan and heat over a medium heat.
3   Add the pulp after 30–60 seconds, then add the tomato quarters and cook for 5–7 minutes.
4   Add the stock cube and passata. Continue to cook over a medium heat for 20 minutes. For about the last 10 minutes of the cooking time, cook the pasta according to the packet instructions.
5   Check the sauce seasoning and add salt and pepper if needed.
6   Serve mixed into the cooked pasta. Place in warmed flasks.

Baked Beans

Baked beans have become something of a British staple. Very few households are without tins of baked beans in their kitchen cupboard, but the taste of home-made beans is much richer and some might say more interesting. It is worth comparing the two by trying this version from time to time.

SERVES 4–6

2 tbsp olive oil

1 onion, diced

3 streaky bacon rashers or handful of lardons, diced

2 x 400g tins of white beans, drained

1 x 400g tin of chopped tomatoes

45g tomato paste

¼ tsp allspice

1 tbsp molasses/treacle

1 tbsp honey

1 tsp sea salt

1   Heat the olive oil in a saucepan and fry the onion and bacon for about 5 minutes until soft.
2   Add the remaining ingredients, bring them to the boil then simmer for 15 minutes.
3   Pop portions into warmed flasks.

Ratatouille

A taste of the Mediterranean. This simple vegetarian dish is delicious as it is or could be added to. Some possible additions include cooked meat, sausages, pulses (cooked) or a scattering of cheese.

SERVES 4–6

2 tbsp olive oil
2 onions, diced
2 garlic cloves, chopped
2 medium-sized courgettes, roughly chopped
1 red pepper, deseeded and chopped
1 orange pepper, deseeded and chopped
1 aubergine, roughly chopped
2 x 400g tins of chopped tomatoes
1 tbsp dried mixed herbs
4 tbsp fresh basil, chopped
Salt and pepper

1 Heat the oil in a pan over a medium heat.
2 Add the onions and garlic and cook for 3–5 minutes, until the onions are translucent.
3 Stir in the courgettes, peppers and aubergine, and cook for a further 5 minutes until lightly coloured.
4 Add the tomatoes and dried mixed herbs, cover and cook over a low heat for 30–35 minutes until the vegetables are tender.
5 Season and sprinkle with chopped basil.
6 Pop into warmed flasks.

Tuna Pasta

Tins of tuna are a real saviour food. They can be used in sandwiches, salads and, as in this dish, with pasta. This is a straightforward pasta dish and is a perfect one to turn to when you've been caught short.

SERVES 2

400g gnocchi (gluten-free optional)
2 tbsp olive oil
1 large garlic clove, chopped
1 x 110g tinned tuna in olive oil, undrained
½ tsp lemon juice
1 tbsp chopped fresh parsley
Parmesan and lemon zest, to serve (optional)
Salt and pepper

1   Boil a salted pot of water for your gnocchi and cook according to the packet instructions.
2   When the pasta is close to being ready, add the oil to a medium-sized frying pan over a medium heat. Once the oil is hot, add the garlic and cook it for 30 seconds.
3   Stir in the tuna, lemon juice and parsley. Let it heat through.
4   Toss the cooked gnocchi into the pan and ensure each piece is evenly coated in the garlicky oil. Season with salt and pepper.
5   Place in warmed flasks. Scatter over the Parmesan and lemon zest.

Sausage and Bean Casserole

A great dish for using up leftover cooked sausages. Complementary flavours from the chorizo, peppers and paprika bring this dish some Mexican flair.

SERVES 2–4

1 tsp olive oil
2 small red onions, chopped
100g chorizo, chopped
1 yellow pepper, diced
1 garlic clove, crushed
1 x 400g tin of low-sugar baked beans
6 cooked sausages, chopped
1 tbsp tomato paste

1   Heat the olive oil in a large pan. Add the onions, chorizo and pepper and sauté for about 5 minutes. Add the garlic and stir for 1 minute.
2   Add the beans, cooked sausages and tomato paste and stir, then cook for about 5 minutes at a simmer until the sausages are cooked through.
3   Place in warmed flasks.

Fishcakes

These fishcakes combine brightly coloured orange sweet potato
with the flakes of freshly baked cod. They are baked and not fried,
making them a healthier option.

MAKES 4 FISHCAKES

240g cod fillet
170g sweet potatoes (without skin), roasted
1 tsp fresh chopped parsley
1 large free-range egg
3 tbsp plain flour (gluten-free or white spelt flour)
1 tsp olive oil
Salt and freshly ground black pepper

1   Preheat the oven to 200°C/Fan 180°C/Gas 6.
2   Bake the cod in the oven for 10 minutes until just cooked. The
    fish should flake apart easily.
3   Mix the fish, roasted sweet potato, parsley and egg together
    until well combined. Season with salt and pepper.
4   Stir in the flour.
5   Shape the mixture into 4 patties, coating them in a little more
    flour to ensure they don't stick to the plate they're resting on
    and set aside to chill in the fridge for 1 hour.
6   Heat the oil in a frying pan and fry the fishcakes until browned
    on each side, then transfer them to an ovenproof dish and bake
    for a further 10 minutes. Serve the fishcakes in warmed flasks
    or leave to cool and serve in the lunchbox with a little salad and
    dressing.

Kofta Meatballs

These little meatballs provide the flavour of the Middle East, yet they're so mild and deliciously aromatic they'll be enjoyed by all ages. They're delicious served alongside some tzatziki or cucumber dill dip.

MAKES ABOUT 15 MEATBALLS

500g minced lamb
1 tbsp minced garlic
1 tsp ground cumin
2 tbsp ground coriander
2 tbsp chopped fresh mint
2 tbsp chopped fresh flat-leaf parsley
½ tsp honey
Salt and pepper

1   Preheat the oven to 200°C/Fan 180°C/Gas 6.
2   Place all ingredients in a mixing bowl and combine everything with your hands.
3   Roll the mixture into table-tennis-sized balls.
4   Place the balls on a baking tray and bake until cooked through. This should take about 12–15 minutes depending on the size of the balls.
5   Place in warmed flasks.

Easy Beef Stew

This is a real winter warmer, a really comforting stew.
Imagine opening your flask at lunchtime to be greeted by this
delightful dish. Yum!

SERVES 4

400g stewing steak
2½ tbsp white spelt or gluten-free flour, seasoned with black pepper
3 tbsp olive oil
2 medium onions, finely chopped
2 garlic cloves, finely chopped
4 medium carrots, peeled and cut into three 3cm pieces
300ml beef stock
1 x 400g tin of chopped tomatoes
2 tsp wholegrain mustard

1   Preheat the oven to 160°C/Fan 140°C/Gas 3.
2   Roll the beef in the seasoned flour.
3   Heat 2 tablespoons of the oil in a large heavy-based, flameproof
    casserole dish and brown the beef in batches.
4   Put the browned beef on to a plate.
5   Add the remaining 1 tablespoon of oil to the casserole dish.
6   Add the onions and cook over a high heat for a couple of
    minutes
7   Turn the heat down and add the garlic. Cover and leave to sweat
    until tender.
8   Once the onions and garlic are soft, add the carrots, stock,
    tomatoes, mustard and the browned beef, then cover and cook
    in the oven for at least 2 hours or until the beef is really tender.
9   Place in warmed flasks.

Mild Chilli Con Carne

As the vegetables in this dish are mostly grated or diced small, the cooking time is reduced and the flavours are released quicker. This is a speedy meal to make and is delicious halfway through the day when you're away from home but want some of your home comforts.

SERVES 4–6

1 tbsp olive oil
1 small onion, finely diced
1 garlic clove, crushed
1 medium carrot, grated
1 small courgette, grated
1 tsp sweet smoked paprika
1 tsp ground coriander
1 tsp ground cumin
½ tsp mild chilli powder
500g beef mince
1 corn on the cob, kernels sliced off the cob
1 x 400g tin of chopped tomatoes
2 tbsp tomato purée
300ml stock (vegetable or beef)
Salt and pepper

1　Heat the oil in a large saucepan. Add the onion, stirring until it starts to soften.
2　Add the garlic, carrot and courgette and fry for another 2–3 minutes.
3　Add the spices and mix well.
4　Add in the beef mince and fry until the meat has browned.
5　Add the sweetcorn kernels, tinned tomatoes, tomato purée and stock and leave to simmer uncovered for 20 minutes. Season to taste.
6　Remove from the heat and place in warmed flasks.

Spaghetti, Bacon and Spinach Frittata

This recipe was 'discovered' when we had a leftover pasta dish one evening and didn't want to waste it. So I heated up the leftovers in a large frying pan and added eggs and cheese, making it into an entirely new dish (as far as the rest of the family were concerned). It went down a storm and we have been eating this regularly ever since.

SERVES 4–6

2 tbsp olive oil
1 onion, chopped
150g unsmoked lardons or chopped, unsmoked bacon
1 garlic clove, crushed
3 ripe plum tomatoes, cut into quarters
2 tbsp tomato purée
½ tsp balsamic vinegar
115g baby spinach
330g leftover cooked spaghetti (gluten-free optional)
6 large eggs, beaten
2 tbsp grated Grana Padano or pecorino cheese
Salt and pepper

1   Heat 1 tablespoon of olive oil in a large saucepan.
2   Add the onion and lardons or bacon and sauté until the onions are soft.
3   Add the garlic, plum tomatoes, tomato purée, balsamic vinegar and season with salt and pepper.
4   Stir then leave to simmer for 5 minutes.
5   Remove the pan from the heat and stir in the baby spinach until wilted.
6   Add the spaghetti to the pan and stir until it is covered in the sauce.
7   Preheat the grill to high.
8   Heat the remaining tablespoon of olive oil in a large frying pan.
9   Add the spaghetti and sauce mix and heat through in the frying pan then add the whisked eggs.

10 Heat until you can see that the bottom of the frittata is cooked, then top with the grated cheese and place under the grill on a high heat.

11 Once the cheese is nicely coloured and the egg is cooked, remove from the grill. This can be placed hot in warmed flasks or left to cool then sliced for lunchboxes.

Green Lentil and Tomato Curry

This is a creamy and mild vegetarian/vegan curry. It's a store cupboard favourite as most of the ingredients are already in the cupboard at home. Great for emergency lunches!

SERVES 2–4

1 tsp olive oil
1 onion, diced
1 tsp grated ginger
1 tsp minced garlic
1 tsp garam masala
½ tsp cumin
¼ tsp turmeric
¼ tsp ground coriander
½ tsp salt
⅛ tsp ground black pepper
½ x 400g tin of chopped tomatoes
1 x 400g tin of green lentils, drained and rinsed
100ml coconut cream or dairy cream

1 Heat the oil in a medium-sized saucepan.
2 Sauté the onion until transparent.
3 Add the ginger and garlic.
4 Sauté for another 2 minutes then add the spices and stir.
5 Add in the salt, pepper and tomatoes, then simmer for 10 minutes or until thickened. Finally, stir in the lentils and coconut cream or cream and check the seasoning. Add more salt if necessary. Serve in warmed flasks.

Vegetable and Lentil Stew

This is warming vegan stew. Very mild in flavour but creamy and satisfying in taste. It's also a great way to use up the last of that packet of red lentils that so often just gets left in the cupboard.

SERVES 1–2

1 tbsp olive oil
1 small onion, diced
1 garlic clove, minced
1 carrot, grated
½ a red pepper, chopped
¼ tsp ground turmeric
½ tsp ground cumin
60g red lentils, rinsed
1½ tbsp tomato paste
4 tbsp coconut cream
Salt and pepper

1   Heat the oil in a small saucepan.
2   Add the onion and sauté until transparent. Stir in the garlic, carrot, red pepper, spices and a little salt and pepper.
3   Add the lentils, tomato paste, coconut cream and just enough water to cover the lentils. Bring to a simmer and simmer for 20 minutes or until the lentils are cooked through. Check the seasoning and serve in warmed flasks.

8 Sauces, Dips and Dressings

The Joy of Sauces, Dips and Dressings

Sauces, dips and dressings are often what really brings ingredients together and makes a dish. Portable lunches are much more interesting and more than the sum of their parts when they are joined by the most suitable dressings and sauces or served with the right dip. They can turn a mundane packed lunch into something your friends, colleagues or school mates will genuinely be jealous of.

Statistically speaking children are much more likely to eat their vegetables if they are served alongside a dip[7]. Let's face it, the same goes for us adults, even if it's something more akin to being 'more likely to eat salad with a dressing' or 'more likely to eat a variety of vegetables in a sauce rather than simply boiled on a plate'. So, it's important to think about some really flavourful sauces, dips and dressings for lunches.

Dressings

The quality of your dressing is only as good as the quality of your ingredients. Better quality oil and vinegars mean better dressings. For example, if a recipe calls for extra virgin olive oil, don't use mild olive oil.

The key to dressings is to properly emulsify the fat and the acid (vinegar or citrus juice). All this means is vigorously whisking the ingredients until the fat breaks down into tiny globules and is evenly spread throughout the oil. Some recipes call for ingredients such as raw honey, mustard or even egg yolk. These are all-natural emulsifiers, which means they naturally help the other ingredients of the dressing come together.

While there are many healthy shop-bought dressings – generally those with real and recognisable ingredients; not the ones with added sweeteners and thickening gums – freshly made dressings are extremely easy to create at home. Freshly made dressings can last for up to a week in an airtight container in the fridge. However, a salad shouldn't be dressed until you are ready to consume it.

[7] https://www.parenthub.com.au/news/parenting-news/dip-dip-hooray-kids-eat-veggies-flavoured-dips/

If you want to make your own home-made salad dressing or dressing for vegetables, follow this simple three-step process:

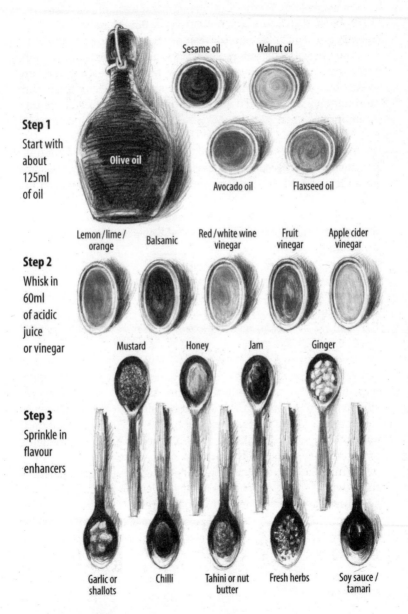

Step 1
Start with about 125ml of oil

Sesame oil

Walnut oil

Olive oil

Avocado oil

Flaxseed oil

Step 2
Whisk in 60ml of acidic juice or vinegar

Lemon / lime / orange

Balsamic

Red / white wine vinegar

Fruit vinegar

Apple cider vinegar

Step 3
Sprinkle in flavour enhancers

Mustard

Honey

Jam

Ginger

Garlic or shallots

Chilli

Tahini or nut butter

Fresh herbs

Soy sauce / tamari

Dips

Dips are easy to transport and are varied in type and flavour. They have so much going for them as lunchbox staples.

A great dip is always flavoursome but balanced. No one ingredient should be discernible over another.

As with dressings, dips are as healthy as the ingredients you put into them, and you can create very creamy dips without adding actual cream or creamy ingredients. Cooked pulses, nuts, seeds and vegetables such as roasted aubergine or sweet potato add natural creaminess to a dip.

Sauces

For packed lunches, sauces that go well with cooked pasta, rice or quinoa are useful. Of course, one of the lunchbox classic pasta sauces is pesto, which combines the earthy flavours of basil with smooth and creamy pine nuts, strong-tasting cheese and good-quality olive oil. However, there are many more possibilities and this chapter will explore some of them.

Recipes

None of the recipes in this chapter take long to prepare. They are designed to be achievable and take up minimal making time but with tasty results.

Rocket and Basil Pesto

A simple change to a classic pesto recipe raises the nutrient profile, increasing zinc, magnesium and B vitamins as well as iron. This pesto is not only delicious in pasta dishes but also in sandwiches and frittatas.

SERVES 4

50g basil leaves, washed and patted dry
25g rocket
75g pecorino or Parmesan cheese, grated
25g pine nuts
1 garlic clove, peeled
100g extra virgin olive oil
Salt and pepper (optional)

1   Simply place all the ingredients except the oil into a food processor and whizz to combine.
2   Add the oil and whizz again. Check the seasoning then serve over pasta, in frittatas or in sandwiches or over salads.

Creamy Butternut Squash Pasta Sauce

Once roasted, butternut squash really sweetens up and takes on a delicate buttery flavour. This sauce is unrecognisable as its starting ingredients, which means it may be a way to encourage those who aren't keen on vegetables in sauces to eat a sauce that's made of vegetables.

SERVES 4–6

300g butternut squash, peeled and cubed (roughly 2cm cubes)
2 small red onions, sliced into sixths
2 garlic cloves, left whole but peeled
1 tsp olive oil
½ tsp salt
45ml cream
30g pecorino or Parmesan cheese, finely grated

1   Preheat the oven to 200°C/Fan 180°C/Gas 6.
2   Place the chopped butternut squash, onions and whole garlic on a small baking tray. Drizzle over 1 teaspoon of olive oil and sprinkle over ½ teaspoon of salt.
3   Bake for 35–40 minutes, tossing the vegetables a couple of times, or until the butternut squash is soft.
4   Leave to cool then process the roasted vegetables with the cream and cheese in a food processor.
5   Add 200ml of water and process again until the sauce reaches the ideal creamy pasta sauce consistency.
6   Warm through and pour over cooked pasta.

Lentil and Tomato Pasta Sauce

Green lentils are a great plant-protein and provide texture and flavour to this flavoursome pasta sauce.

1 tsp olive oil
1 onion, diced
1 garlic clove, crushed
1 x 400g tin of chopped tomatoes
100ml vegetable stock
1 x 400g green lentils, drained and rinsed
Salt and pepper

1   Heat the oil in a medium saucepan.
2   Sauté the onion until it becomes transparent then add the garlic and stir for 1 minute.
3   Add the tinned tomatoes, vegetable stock and salt and pepper. Simmer uncovered for 10 minutes or until thickened.
4   Add the lentils and stir. Turn off the heat and allow the lentils to heat through.
5   Serve over cooked pasta.

Classic Tomato Sauce

This is an extremely simple way to create a classic tomato pasta sauce from very few ingredients. In fact, these might just be the ingredients left in the vegetable drawer of your fridge at the end of the week, so it's a great way to use up leftovers. You could add other leftover cooked vegetables towards the end of the recipe to create an even more nutrient-dense pasta sauce.

SERVES 2–4

1 tbsp olive oil
1 onion, chopped
1 x 400g carton of chopped tomatoes in tomato juice
½ vegetable stock cube
½ tsp garlic granules
1 tsp dried oregano

1   Heat the olive oil in a medium saucepan.
2   Add the onion and sauté for about 5 minutes.
3   Add about 2 tablespoons of the tomatoes in tomato juice, the stock cube, the garlic granules and oregano.
4   Once the tomatoes have thickened add another 2 tablespoons of tomatoes in juice.
5   Repeat this one more time in order to make the onions really soft and 'jammy'.
6   Then add the rest of the tomatoes in juice and heat through.
7   Leave to cool then place in a food processor and process to the desired consistency. Ideally thick but not chunky.
8   It is now ready to serve on freshly cooked pasta or courgetti.

Beetroot Hummus

A slightly earthier take on a classic hummus. This is a very pink dip and might appeal to some for this reason. It is sweeter in taste and works well with a crumble of feta cheese on top.

SERVES 4–6

1 x 400g can of chickpeas in water, drained and rinsed
1 x 250g pack of cooked beetroot, drained and roughly chopped
2 tbsp extra virgin olive oil
1 tbsp tahini
1 tbsp apple cider vinegar
1 garlic clove, peeled
Salt and pepper

1   Put all the ingredients into a food processor with 1 tablespoon of water and process at full speed. Season to taste. That's it!

Serving suggestion: Add 75g of crumbled feta on top of the dip.

Red Pepper Hummus

Brightly coloured, roasted peppers bring colour, texture and great flavour to this delicious hummus. With a little salt and smoked paprika for serving, this hummus is a great variation on a standard hummus and a good introduction to those new to hummus, too.

SERVES 4–6

1 x 400g tin of chickpeas, drained and rinsed
About ½ a 290g jar of roasted red peppers, drained
2 tbsp tahini or nut/seed butter
1 garlic clove, minced
1 tbsp olive oil
½ tsp salt
½ tsp ground cumin
A pinch of sweet smoked paprika, to serve
Salt and pepper

1 Put all the ingredients, except the paprika, in a food processor and process until smooth.
2 Check the seasoning and sprinkle the paprika over the top. Serve with crackers or chopped vegetable batons in your lunchbox.

Aubergine Tahini Dip

When aubergine is baked, it turns into a buttery consistency
that only adds to the deliciousness of this creamy Middle
East-inspired dip.

2 medium aubergines, sliced into 2cm discs
3 tbsp olive oil
A good pinch of sea salt
1 heaped tsp tahini
Juice of ½ lemon
Honey, to taste

1   Preheat the oven to 200°C/Fan 180°C/Gas 6.
2   Lay the slices of aubergine on 2 baking sheets.
3   Roast the aubergines with 2 tbsp of olive oil drizzled evenly
    over the top and sprinkled with sea salt for 25 minutes, turning
    frequently. (Note: they soak up a lot of oil. This is fine as it will
    add to the velvety texture of the dip.)
4   Leave to cool then place the roasted aubergines, tahini and
    lemon juice into your food processor and process. You may need
    to add another tablespoon of oil to get the correct, smooth
    consistency. When smooth, add ½ a teaspoon of honey. Process
    again and adjust the seasoning until you are satisfied with the
    flavour.
5   Serve with cucumber batons or pitta chips.

Pea and Mint Dip

A classic combination of pea and mint pairs up to create this flavoursome, refreshing dip.

<u>SERVES 4–6</u>

300g fresh peas, or frozen peas, defrosted (ideally petit pois, which are tender and sweet)
4 tbsp fresh mint, finely chopped
140g natural yogurt
15g pecorino cheese
Juice of ½ lemon
Salt and pepper

1   Place the peas and mint in a food processor and process until you have a paste-like consistency.
2   In another bowl, add the natural yogurt, pecorino cheese, lemon juice and salt and pepper and mix well. Add the pea and mint mixture and stir thoroughly until all the ingredients are combined.
3   Taste and adjust the seasoning as required.

Cucumber and Onion Raita

This is a delicious dish to have alongside some of the curries in this book. It's also great simply as a dip for other vegetables or for crispbreads or crackers.

SERVES 2–4

300g Greek yogurt
¼ large cucumber, peeled, deseeded and either finely chopped or grated
(depending on your preference texturally)
¼ red onion, grated
½ tsp garam masala
1 tbsp chopped mint
A pinch of salt

1   Mix all the ingredients in a bowl, then chill in the fridge overnight before serving.

Peanut Korma Curry Dip

This is a rich and peanutty taste of Asia!

SERVES 2

½ tsp garlic and ginger paste, or ¼ tsp of each grated
½ tsp cumin
¼ tsp coriander
¼ tsp turmeric
1 tsp soy sauce or tamari
1 tbsp peanut butter
1 tsp honey
80g coconut cream

1   Mix the ingredients together in a small saucepan. Heat gently until combined. Leave to cool then serve with vegetables.

Almond Butter Dipping Sauce

If you prefer almonds and a less creamy dip then this dipping sauce is really easy to make and packs a flavour punch. It's simply a case of preparing a few ingredients and stirring them together in a small bowl. So easy!

SERVES 2

1 tsp grated ginger
1 small garlic clove, grated
Juice of ½ orange
Juice of ½ lime
1 tbsp almond butter
1 tbsp tamari
1 tsp honey

1   Mix all the ingredients together in a small bowl or ramekin with 1 tablespoon of water and serve.

Smoked Mackerel Pâté

Although most people think they get sufficient omega 3 from a balanced diet, in fact 98 per cent of people are deficient[8]. Mackerel is a great source of omega 3 yet few people love the taste, especially children. However, it's my observation that more people enjoy smoked mackerel pâté than enjoy mackerel itself. This creamier fish pâté is a real crowd-pleaser. It's perfect with crackers or sweet pepper fingers.

SERVES 2–4

180g skinless, boneless smoked mackerel fillets (I tend to buy 240g pack with skin on and then peel and take out any bones)
100g cream cheese
Zest and juice of ½ lemon
2 tsp horseradish sauce
Sprinkling of sea salt and freshly ground black pepper

1   Flake the smoked mackerel into small pieces with your fingers or a fork and place in a large bowl with the other ingredients.
2   Mix together well with a fork.
3   Season to taste. Remember that smoked fish is naturally salty though, so you may not need to add any salt, just pepper.

Note: Tinned salmon could be used instead of the mackerel. You'll need a 213g tin, drained of any liquid then used in exactly the same way as the mackerel.

[8] [1] Thuppal, S.V.; von Schacky, C.; Harris, W.S.; Sherif, K.D.; Denby, N.; Steinbaum, S.R.; Haycock, B.; Bailey, R.L. Discrepancy between Knowledge and Perceptions of Dietary Omega-3 Fatty Acid Intake Compared with the Omega-3 Index. *Nutrients* 2017, *9*, 930.

Honey and Mustard Dressing

This is a great salad dressing to make at the start of the week. It goes well with so many salads and really a salad is not a true salad until it has been dressed properly.

SERVES 6

125g plain Greek yogurt
60ml extra-virgin olive oil
2 tbsp Dijon mustard
3 tbsp raw honey
2 tbsp lemon juice
2 tbsp apple cider vinegar
1 garlic clove, minced
½ teaspoon fine sea salt
Freshly ground black pepper

1   Combine all the ingredients in a medium bowl.
2   Whisk until blended.
3   Check the seasoning and season with additional pepper if necessary.
4   This dressing is intentionally bold, but if it tastes too tart for your liking, whisk in another tablespoon of honey.
5   Store the leftover salad dressing covered in the fridge for 10–14 days.

9 The 'Crunch' Factor

Our Love of Crunchy Snacks

Crisps are the second most common component in a packed lunch. In fact, British people eat their way through approximately 150 bags of crisps each per year. Why? Convenience, taste and possibly the multi-million pound advertising and marketing campaigns that mean they are ever present in our consciousness! They're a very attractive snack proposition. They come in their own portion-sized packs (unless we are lured into purchasing 'grab bags', which tend to be larger than the standard bag and subsequently more like a meal in energy terms but not in terms of any other nutrients); they hit the spot meeting our natural desire for salt and fat, and sometimes even sugar; and they crunch. Humans love crunchy, noisy snacks, because the noise helps us identify what it is we're consuming. Depending on the snack, the noise can reach 63 decibels (dB). For context, normal conversations are around 60 decibels, rustling leaves are 20 decibels. This seems to add another layer of pleasure and enjoyment to these not-so-healthy snacks.

Why Not Crisps?

Given our love of these noisy, crunchy snacks I am sorry to be the bearer of some frustrating news. From a nutritional standpoint there's not a huge amount going for them. They often contain added flavours, preservatives, artificial colours and many also now contain added sugars. Crisps conform very well to the stereotype of what is known as the 'bliss point' of food. The bliss point is a recognised combination of sugar, salt and fat that makes sure we are unable to stop eating that food.

From an evolutionary perspective we are conditioned to seek out these three tastes in a precise ratio that links to the brain's pleasure zones. Finding these tastes in these ratios ensured our survival when food was scarce. However, these days we have too much sugar and often salt too in our diet and yet our brains are hard-wired to seek out these pleasure-giving tastes. That makes it difficult to move away from our favourite snacks but there are some healthier, more natural alternatives that are health-giving and don't add to an already overloaded (with sugar and salt) body.

Crisp Alternatives

Knowing that our desire for salty, crunchy, snack-type foods is a natural thing it's reassuring to know that there are both shop-bought healthier alternatives and also some that we can make at home ourselves.

Shop-bought Crisp Alternatives

If you really don't want to make anything at home to take to work or pack for school as a crisp alternative, then these would be the better shop-bought options available:

- Plain or salted popcorn
- Lightly salted tortilla chips
- Plantain chips
- Root vegetable crisps (some are baked, some are fried. Baked are obviously better for you but fried shouldn't be off limits, especially when compared to fried crisps)
- Salted coconut curls
- Seaweed thins
- Dried apple rings
- Baked/roasted, lightly salted broad beans
- Baked/roasted, lightly salted yellow/green peas
- Roasted seeds
- Nuts

Recipes

If you want to take control of the crisp element of your lunch and make your own crunchy snacks then the following recipes will help.

Kale Chips

They sound super-healthy but more importantly they're super-easy to make with the added benefit of being healthy too. Even those who don't like kale or are unwilling to try it in other forms seem to be converted by these crispy kale chips.

MAKES 4 PORTIONS

200g kale, thick stems removed and rinsed well in water
½ tsp extra-virgin olive oil
Sea salt, to serve (optional)

1   Preheat the oven to 140°C/Fan 120°C/Gas 1.
2   Pat the kale dry.
3   Tear it into similar-sized pieces and toss together with the olive oil until well coated.
4   Spread the kale out over 2 baking trays, making sure the leaves aren't touching each other.
5   Cook for 15 minutes, then turn and cook for a further 15 minutes until crisp.
6   Remove from the oven and scatter with a little sea salt, if you like.

Baked Pitta Chips

These are so simple to make and an alternative way to use pittas in a lunchbox. They're fantastic dipped into soup or creamy dips and they really do have the crunch-factor.

SERVES 4

4 organic round wholegrain pitta breads
2 tbsp olive oil
1½ tsp garlic granules
1½ tsp dried oregano

1   Preheat the oven to 200°C/Fan 180°C/Gas 6.
2   Cut the pittas into quarters.
3   Lay the quarters on a baking sheet. Drizzle over the oil, sprinkle with the garlic granules and oregano.
4   Bake for 8–10 minutes until crisp and browned at the edges.
5   Leave to cool before serving in your lunchbox.

Seeded Crackers

With increased focus on real foods, you'll find that crackers can become a minefield of additional ingredients with many made using cheaper flours to bulk them out and gums to bind them. If you want naturally protein-rich crackers made from simple ingredients these meet the mark. They're made from nuts, chia and flaxseeds, meaning they're rich in fibre and they taste amazing.

MAKES ABOUT 30 CRACKERS

180g almonds or walnuts
50g flaxseeds
50g chia seeds
½ tsp dried thyme
½ tsp dried oregano
¼ tsp bicarbonate of soda
½ tsp salt
1 tbsp coconut oil
1 tbsp warm water
1 large egg or 1 flax egg (1 tbsp ground flaxseeds mixed with 3 tbsp warm water and left to settle for 10 minutes)

1   Preheat the oven to 200°C/Fan 180°C/Gas 6.
2   Grind the almonds or walnuts, flaxseeds and chia seeds in a food processor until you have a flour consistency.
3   Add the herbs, bicarbonate, salt, oil, warm water and egg. Combine again in the food processor to form a dough.
4   Roll out the dough between 2 pieces of baking parchment to about 2mm thick. Remove the top sheet of baking parchment and score 'finger' crackers into the dough.
5   Place the dough with the sheet of baking parchment still underneath it on to a baking tray. Bake for 20 minutes until cooked through.
6   Using a knife, ensure each cracker is separate from each other.
7   Leave to cool before serving. Store in an airtight container.

Flax Crackers

Flax seeds have a long history of providing both a nutritious fibre-rich and protein-rich food source. These crunchy crackers will keep you full for hours. They are best served with dips and soups.

MAKES 20

180g ground flaxseeds
2 tbsp sunflower seeds
1 tbsp pumpkin seeds
½ tsp salt
½ tsp mixed herbs

1   Preheat the oven to 200°C/Fan 180°C/Gas 6.
2   Line a baking sheet with greaseproof paper.
3   Combine the flaxseeds and 125ml of water in a bowl.
4   Once a dough is starting to form, add the sunflower and pumpkin seeds and ensure they are evenly distributed throughout the dough. Push the dough onto the baking sheet and flatten until even and about ½cm thick.
5   Sprinkle over the salt and herbs.
6   Score out 20 crackers then bake for 20–30 minutes or until browned around the edges.
7   Leave to cool before serving. Store in an airtight container.

Oatcakes

Not so much cakes as coarse crackers. These are traditionally from Scotland where oats were so widely consumed that Samuel Johnson famously stated in his 1755 dictionary that oats are 'A grain, which in England is generally given to horses, but in Scotland supports the people.' Lord Elibank was said to have retorted: 'Yes, and where else will you see such horses and such men?'

MAKES ABOUT 20 (NUMBER VARIES ACCORDING TO HOW THICK YOU MAKE THEM)

250g porridge oats, ground/processed to a flour, plus a little extra for rolling
½ teaspoon bicarbonate of soda
A pinch of salt
25g butter, melted
150ml hot water

1   Preheat the oven to 200°C/Fan 180°C/Gas 6.
2   Put the oat flour in a large bowl.
3   Add the bicarbonate of soda and the salt.
4   Add the butter and hot water.
5   Stir well with a wooden spoon.
6   Finally, use your hands to bring the soft paste together.
7   Sprinkle your work surface with a little extra oat flour.
8   Roll out the dough – the thickness is up to you, depending on whether you like thin or thick oatcakes.
9   Use a cookie cutter to mark out the rounds.
10 Place them on a baking tray.
11 Bake in the oven for up to 15 minutes.
12 Remove them from oven and allow to cool a little.
13 Place on a wire rack to cool completely.
14 The oatcakes will keep in an airtight container for a few days.

Oaty Cheese Biscuits

A cheesy version of an oatcake for those that love cheese and want something a little more savoury.

MAKES ABOUT 10 BISCUITS

50g oat flour or oats, processed to a flour using a food processor
50g spelt flour or gluten-free plain flour, plus a little extra for rolling
A pinch of salt
60g butter, plus extra for greasing
80g Cheddar cheese, grated
2 tbsp cold water

1   Preheat the oven to 200°C/Fan 180°C/Gas 6.
2   Combine the flours with the salt and butter using your fingertips.
3   Add the grated cheese and the cold water.
4   Mix to form a dough. Roll out on to a floured board to about 1.5cm thick.
5   Cut any shapes you want.
6   Grease 2 baking trays with a little extra butter.
7   Place the biscuits on to the trays and bake in the oven for 20 minutes.
8   Remove and leave to cool.

Crispy Roasted Cauliflower

This is a simple but delicious way to enjoy this incredibly versatile vegetable. Once roasted, the natural sugars in the cauliflower come to the fore, making this a tasty option even for those who don't like cauliflower served in the more traditional ways. Try it before you deny it.

SERVES 4

1 cauliflower head
Olive oil
½ tsp salt

1   Preheat the oven to 200°C/Fan 180°C/Gas 6.
2   Cut the cauliflower crossways into 2cm-thick slices. Set aside.
3   Coat a baking sheet with olive oil.
4   Place the cauliflower slices on to the prepared baking sheet in a single layer and drizzle over a little oil. Season with salt.
5   Roast in the preheated oven for about 30 minutes, or until browned and crisp. Toss the cauliflower once during cooking.
6   Serve warm or cold in your lunchbox.

Spicy Roasted Chickpeas

Chickpeas are incredibly versatile, and this snack really shows
them off at their best. These tasty, crunchy bites really give the
impression of eating something snacky and yet they're adding
valuable nutrients with every bite.

SERVES 4–6

1 x 400g can of chickpeas, drained and rinsed
1 tbsp olive oil
¼ tsp chilli powder
¼ tsp sweet smoked paprika
½ tsp dried thyme leaves
⅓ tsp salt

1   Preheat the oven to 190°C/Fan 170°C/Gas 5.
2   Spread the chickpeas into a single layer on a baking sheet.
3   Bake for 30 minutes, shaking the pan every now and then.
4   Remove the chickpeas from the oven and carefully place the hot
    chickpeas into a bowl along with the olive oil, chilli powder,
    paprika, thyme and salt.
5   Toss well to coat the chickpeas evenly.
6   Spread the seasoned chickpeas back on to the baking sheet and
    return to the oven for another 10–15 minutes until they are
    golden and crispy.
7   Leave to cool before serving.

Roasted Beetroot and Salt Crisps

These are a far more interesting than the traditional potato-based crisp. They have a really deep, earthy and slightly sweet flavour brought to life by the addition of a little salt. They become beautifully crispy at the edges and crispier in the middle the longer you bake them. They are delicious with a tzatziki-style dip or as part of a salad.

SERVES 3–4 AS A VEGETABLE PORTION IN A LUNCHBOX

2 beetroots, peeled and sliced ½cm thick
1 tbsp olive oil
Sea salt

1   Preheat the oven to 220°C/Fan 200°C/Gas 7.
2   Grease and line a baking sheet with greaseproof paper.
3   Place the beetroot slices in a bowl, add the oil and season with salt, then mix together to ensure each beetroot slice is covered.
4   Place the beetroot slices on the baking sheet and put them in the oven.
5   Cook for 15 minutes then flip the slices over and place them back in the oven for another 15 minutes, until crispy.

Sweet and Spicy Seeds

A simple mix of seeds with some delicious salt and sweet flavours.
These can be eaten just as they are or they can be added to the top of
dips or salads for extra crunch and texture.

SERVES 2–4

125g mixed seeds (sunflower, pumpkin, poppy)
½ tsp olive oil
¼ tsp sweet smoked paprika
½ tsp soy sauce or tamari
½ tsp maple syrup

1 Preheat the oven to 200°C/Fan 180°C/Gas 6.
2 In a bowl, combine the oil, paprika, soy sauce or tamari and
   maple syrup. Toss the seeds to coat.
3 Lay the seeds flat on a lined baking sheet in a single layer.
4 Bake for 7–10 minutes until golden.
5 Leave to cool then pack into a container with a lid for lunch.

Popcorn

Popcorn is a simple and ideal wholefood addition to a lunchbox but many people find it hard to cook. This method is super-easy and hard to get wrong.

SERVES 6

2 tbsp coconut oil
50g popcorn kernels
Salt

1   Heat the oil in a large, sturdy saucepan.
2   Add just a couple of popcorn kernels to the pan.
3   Once they pop, add the others.
4   Add the lid and shake the pan. Keep shaking as the kernels start to pop.
5   Once the popping slows significantly, remove the pan from the heat and keep shaking until the last kernel has popped. Take the lid off and pour the contents into a bowl.
6   Sprinkle salt over the popcorn to taste.

Cheesy Polenta Fingers

Polenta is basically cornmeal, i.e. ground corn. Traditional polenta takes a lot of preparation, stirring and standing over a pot for ages. Instant polenta means the work has already been done for you. These little polenta fingers are deliciously cheesy, and the flavours of cheese and herbs combine to bring this savoury snack to life.

MAKES 30–35 POLENTA CHIPS

Olive oil, for greasing, plus 1–2 tbsp, for baking
220g fine (instant) polenta
110g mature Cheddar cheese, finely grated
1 tbsp salted butter
Salt and pepper

1   Brush the inside of a 20 x 20cm roasting pan with olive oil.
2   Bring 1 litre of water to a rolling boil in a large saucepan.
3   Steadily sprinkle in the instant polenta and stir/whisk constantly until it starts to thicken significantly. Remove from heat and stir in the Cheddar cheese and butter.
4   Have a taste and add salt if needed and black pepper to your taste.
5   Pour the polenta into the prepared roasting pan. Leave to cool then place in the fridge for at least 3 hours.
6   Turn out the block of polenta on to a chopping board and use a large knife to slice it into thick batons about 2 x 5cm.
7   Preheat the oven to 210°C/Fan 190°C/Gas 6½.
8   Pour about 1–2 tablespoons of olive oil into a baking tray. Heat this for about 5 minutes in the oven then carefully add the batons with some salt over the top. Turn the batons in the hot oil then place in the oven and bake for 30 minutes or until golden and crispy on the outside.
9   These can be served warm or cold in your lunchbox.

Halloumi (Baked) Fries

Halloumi has a rare texture for a cheese. Some claim it makes a squeaky sound when they eat it. These cheesy fingers are packed full of flavour and texture. Whether you find them squeaky or not, you're sure to enjoy these unique 'fries'.

MAKES ABOUT 20

250g halloumi cheese
¼ ½ tsp sweet smoked paprika, to taste
40g coconut flour
1 large egg

1 Preheat the oven to 180°C/Fan 160°C/Gas 4.
2 Line a baking tray with greaseproof paper.
3 Slice the halloumi into 2cm sticks.
4 Mix the paprika and coconut flour in a bowl. Coat the halloumi sticks in the flour mix.
5 Crack open the egg in a bowl and whisk with a fork.
6 Dip the coated halloumi into the egg, shake off any excess then carefully roll again in the remaining paprika and coconut flour mix. Place the coated halloumi sticks on to the prepared baking tray.
7 Bake for 17–18 minutes, turning once during cooking. They should be golden brown and crunchy on the outside. Cool then serve in your lunchbox.

Cheese Straws

These grain-free cheese straws are perfect for those wanting a
lower carbohydrate-based cheese straw and/or for those who
cannot tolerate grains. They're a great high-protein, lower-carb
lunchbox addition.

MAKES ABOUT 25

120g ground almonds, plus extra for rolling
1 heaped tsp psyllium husk
150g mature Cheddar cheese, very finely grated
1 egg
2 tbsp extra virgin olive oil, plus extra for greasing

1 Preheat the oven to 200°C/Fan 180°C/Gas 6.
2 In a bowl, mix together the ground almonds and psyllium, then
   add the finely grated Cheddar and stir.
3 Add the egg and the oil and bring everything together with your
   hands. Using some more ground almonds, roll the dough out to
   about ½cm thick and cut 5cm long fingers.
4 Lay these on to a greased and lined baking sheet or 2 and bake
   for 15 minutes.
5 Leave to cool completely before serving in your lunchbox.

One-ingredient Cheese Crackers

These are easy to make and delicious to eat. What's not to like about
a one-ingredient recipe? You must use a silicone cover on your
baking tray or some greaseproof paper to ensure you can actually
get the crisps off the sheet at the end of cooking.

MAKES ABOUT 40

225g Cheddar cheese, finely grated

1. Preheat the oven to 200°C/Fan 180°C/Gas 6.
2. Cover a large baking sheet with a silicone baking sheet or with greaseproof paper.
3. Put small piles of the cheese at even intervals on the sheet. Allow a little room for them to spread out while cooking.
4. Bake for 9 minutes. They should be golden brown and almost stiff (not bendy).
5. Cool then peel them off and place in your lunchbox.

Protein Tortillas

This recipe comes from my colleague Jen Roach from Fearless in the Kitchen. Jen and I run workshops from her cookery school in Berkshire . These tortillas are always a hit at our co-run events. Pea flour is high in protein and B vitamins as well as being a source of prebiotic fibre. It has 25 per cent more protein than wheat flour. If you don't have yellow pea flour then you can simply substitute chickpea flour in this recipe.

MAKES 8–10, DEPENDING ON FRYING PAN SIZE

400g yellow pea flour
3 tbsp olive oil, plus extra for frying
Pinch of salt and pepper

1 Tip the pea flour, salt and pepper into a bowl. Whisk in 3 tablespoons of oil, 400ml of water and then let it sit, covered, for 15 minutes.
2 Preheat the oven to 200°C/Fan 180°C/Gas 6.
3 Grease a small frying pan and make sure the pan is hot before tipping in enough batter to lightly coat the pan (the pan needs to be hot to start with or your batter will stick).
4 Once the batter is in the pan, tilt the pan so it coats the base evenly and turn the heat to medium.
5 Cook for 2–3 minutes on one side. When bubbles form on the surface and the batter starts to brown, flip the tortilla over and cook for a minute.
6 Remove the tortilla from the pan and set it aside under a tea towel to keep warm.
7 Ensure there's a light coating of oil in the pan before you add the next set of batter.
8 Repeat with the remaining batter.
9 Prepare a baking tray with a light coating of olive oil
10 Cut the cooked tortillas into triangles or squares.
11 Lay them out in a single layer. Sprinkle with salt.
12 Bake for 15 minutes. (The time will depend on the thickness of the tortilla. It's worth cooking for slightly longer so the crackers are crisp.)

Courgette Chips

Courgettes seem distinctly underrated. Perhaps they need just a little added flavour to elevate them to the heights of more favoured vegetables. This recipe uses strongly flavoured cheese to provide that flavour lift.

2 eggs
100g Parmesan or pecorino, finely grated
20g dried breadcrumbs (gluten-free optional)
2 courgettes (about 400–500g in total), sliced into thick fingers, about 5cm long

1   Preheat the oven to 220°C/Fan 200°C/Gas Mark 7.
2   Beat the eggs and place them in a bowl.
3   Combine the cheese and breadcrumbs.
4   Dip the courgette fingers in the eggs then into the bowl with the cheese and breadcrumbs.
5   Place on a baking sheet covered with greaseproof paper or silicone and bake for 15 minutes. They should be golden brown and crisp.
6   Leave to cool before serving in your lunchbox.

10 Where's My Yogurt?

What Happened to Healthy Yogurt?

The food industry has a reputation for taking what was once a healthy food and turning it into processed junk food and this is exactly what has happened to most yogurts. In recent years, yogurts have become less and less like the healthy food they once were and more like a full-on sugar-loaded dessert, with chocolate balls and even sweets provided to tip into an already sweetened yogurt.

Yet, Yogurt Can Be Healthy

The reality is that yogurt can be an immensely healthy food. It is one of the oldest and most popular fermented foods worldwide. By fermented food we mean a food that provides health benefits as a result of the 'good' bacteria present, which multiply to give yogurt its distinctive tangy flavour. Not only do the bacteria provide health benefits but yogurt also provides protein and calcium, two of the six components of a nutritionally balanced lunchtime meal.

Probiotics

In the supermarket aisle dedicated to yogurts you will find lots of yogurt-like products alongside the genuine, traditional product. The first thing you'll notice in a healthy, traditional yogurt and not a yogurt-like product is that it contains probiotic bacteria. Pro means 'for' and biotic means 'life'. When we eat probiotic bacteria, they can live on in our gut and become part of our gut flora – a community of beneficial microbes. These bacteria have been linked to improved digestion, but studies have also shown that they may be able to improve many other body systems and ailments including skin health, mental health, weight management as well as reducing our propensity to suffer from lifestyle-related diseases.

Expect to see names such as Bifidobacterium Bifidum, Bifidobacterium Animalis Lactis, Lactobacillus Bulgaricus, Streptococcus Thermophilus, Lactobacillus Acidophilus and Lactobacillus Casei, Lactobacillus Rhamnosus, Lactobacillus Plantarum, Lactococcus Lactis, listed on the label. It is important to seek out these bacteria on the labels of yogurts, as a product without beneficial bacteria can still be called a yogurt even though it doesn't contain probiotic bacteria. Another advantage of buying yogurts made in the traditional way is that the probiotic bacteria ferment and break down the lactose into lactic acid. This makes real yogurt a lower lactose product, which for those with a lactose intolerance – and that's about 65 per cent of the general population – is helpful.

Natural Sugars

Some yogurts have as much as five teaspoonfuls of sugar in them. That's equivalent to three scoops of some ice creams. That's when these yogurt-like desserts start to become more like sugar-laden puddings than contributors to health. So, the second thing you should look for in a healthier yogurt is less than 10g of sugar per 100g of product. Try also to compare serving size and be realistic about what would be served in a lunchbox. Most individual yogurts are packed in 150g pots. The sugar content is not always obvious on the pot as most often calculations are made per 100g of product. A 150g pot of yogurt might have a label telling you it contains 12g of sugar per 100g of product. That means that the 150g pot contains 18g of sugar, which equates to 4½ teaspoons.

Be aware of added sweeteners in yogurts though. As we become more sugar aware so manufacturers are becoming smarter and reducing the added refined sugars, but in their place they're adding artificial sweeteners. Although artificial sweeteners have been used in food products for many years, you don't need to look far to find someone who has had an adverse reaction to one or more of them. Furthermore, evidence is now emerging that excessive consumption of artificial sweeteners disrupts the microbiome, upsetting the balance of bacteria in the gut. This could undo all of those health benefits mentioned above, but ironically, it may also lead to weight gain. So, when looking at yogurt labels, read the ingredients labels too and be aware of added artificial sweeteners.

Actual Fruit

Pictures of actual fruit on the packaging do not necessarily mean you'll find fruit in a pot of yogurt. While some refer to the yogurt being fruit-flavoured it may be just that: flavour has been added to make it taste like the fruit/s depicted on the packaging. Furthermore, fruit compotes mentioned on the description of the yogurt on the packaging or pot itself may also be concentrated sugars with little added fruit. Check the ingredients label. Ideally, the fruit depicted on the outside of the yogurt will feature in the ingredients list. Furthermore, the sweetness in the yogurt should ideally come from fruit with little or no added sugars.

Do We Need Thickening Agents?

Thickening agents and gums are often added to yogurts to give them viscosity without changing the taste of the yogurt. Their purpose is to absorb fluid and in so doing thicken that fluid. These are not overtly unhealthy, but in a traditional yogurt made according to a traditional recipe they should not be necessary because thickness is the result of the traditional yogurt-making method – in which the yogurt is strained and fermented.

To summarise, the attributes you want to look for in an ideal yogurt are:

- Some probiotic bacteria named on the label
- 10g of sugar per 100g product or less
- Contains sugar from fruit only, not refined sugar
- No artificial sweeteners
- Some real fruit if it is a fruit yogurt
- No added thickeners
- No added colours, flavours or preservatives

There are plenty of more natural, real food-based yogurts and yogurt-like desserts on the market. Some of the better shop-bought options include:

- Plain Greek yogurt
- Greek yogurt (unsweetened) and honey
- Bircher muesli yogurts (check for added sugars)
- Chia puddings
- Coconut yogurt (made from coconut milk and using probiotic bacteria)
- Almond milk-based yogurts

Recipes

If you are looking for some home-made options that put you in control of how much fruit, sugar and how thick your dessert is, or if yogurt is not your thing but you want an alternative pudding in your lunchbox, then check out the following recipes.

Apple and Orange Compote for Yogurt

A delicious apple and orange compote, flavoured with a touch of cinnamon. The sweetness comes only from fruit and the flavour combination works wonderfully well over yogurt.

MAKES 4–6 PORTIONS

3 eating apples, thickly sliced or wedged (using a wedger)
150ml orange juice
Pinch of cinnamon

1   Put the apples into a small saucepan and pour over the orange juice, then add the pinch of cinnamon.
2   Simmer for 10 minutes until the apples are soft.
3   Cool slightly then, using a food processor, blend the compote.
4   Serve over yogurt.

Berry Coulis for Yogurt

If you prefer the taste of summer fruits to that of apple and cinnamon, then this berry coulis is a really simple way to add great flavour to natural yogurt.

MAKES 4–6 PORTIONS

350g frozen berries
1–2 tbsp honey, to taste
½ tsp vanilla extract

1   Put the berries in a small pan with 60ml of water.
2   When the berries begin to soften, add the honey and vanilla. Start with 1 tablespoon of honey and add more depending on the amount of sweetness you like.
3   Cook until the fruit is very soft. Let everything cool slightly then, using a blender, blend until puréed.
4   Serve over yogurt.

Simple Fruit Purée

If the previous recipe seems like too many steps, then this one will be right up your street. It's a one-ingredient recipe. These purées, whatever fruit you choose, can be stirred into thick Greek yogurt to create a delicious fruit-flavoured yogurt without 'bits'.

MAKES 4–6 PORTIONS

420–435g tinned fruit in fruit juice

1. Simply process the contents of the tin in a food processor to form a purée.
2. Serve this over or stirred through thick and creamy Greek yogurt.

Blueberry Chia Pudding

When chia seeds are soaked in any kind of liquid, they become jelly-like. This dessert benefits from their magic properties and combines antioxidant-rich berries and pomegranate seeds.

SERVES 1–2

90g frozen blueberries
160ml milk (non-dairy optional)
1 tsp maple syrup, to taste
3 tbsp chia seeds
2 tbsp pomegranate seeds, to serve

1   Place the blueberries in your blender along with the milk and maple syrup. Blend on high until smooth.
2   Transfer to a bowl and mix in the chia seeds. Cover and store in the fridge overnight to set.
3   Place in lunchbox containers.
4   Top with pomegranate seeds.

Chia Chocolate Pudding

This recipe combines the higher protein and fibre benefits of chia to create a filling and nutritious chocolatey dessert. Once again, the chia seeds work their jelly-like magic once left to soak overnight.

MAKES 2

250ml milk (non-dairy optional)
1 tbsp cocoa powder
1 tbsp maple syrup (or less depending on your preference)
Pinch of cinnamon
4 tbsp chia seeds
1 small ripe banana, to serve
Dark chocolate, grated, to serve

1   Mix the milk, cocoa powder, maple syrup and cinnamon together in a bowl and stir to combine.
2   Add the chia seeds and stir until well combined.
3   Divide the mixture into lunchbox pots, put on the lids and refrigerate overnight. Give the pots one last shake or stir before you go to bed.
4   During this time, the liquid will be absorbed, and the magic will happen. The pudding will form a jelly-like consistency.
5   Stir in the chopped banana to stop it from going brown and top with grated dark chocolate. Replace the lids on the pots.

Chia Oat Pudding

Using the magic gelling properties of chia seeds once more but combining them with wholesome oats, vanilla, yogurt and honey makes for a very satisfying alternative to a simple yogurt.

SERVES 2–4

50g porridge oats (gluten-free optional)
200ml milk (non-dairy optional)
½ tsp vanilla extract
2 heaped tbsp Greek yogurt
25g chia seeds
½ tsp raw honey or maple syrup

1   Mix the ingredients together and leave to soak overnight.
2   The following day, divide the pudding into lunch containers and top with some fruit.

Serving suggestion: Pomegranate seeds, frozen berries, fresh berries or even some apple or other fruit-based compote.

Cheat's Bircher Muesli

A quick and nutritious way to make and enjoy a substantial oat and yogurt-based dessert with added, beneficial fruit.

SERVES 2–4

50g oats (gluten-free optional)
40g apple purée
20ml apple juice
20ml milk (non dairy optional)
20g frozen berries
50g natural yogurt

To serve
More yogurt, nuts or seeds and fresh fruit

1 Place the ingredients in a large bowl. Stir then soak overnight.
2 The following morning, make up portions and serve with yogurt, nuts/seeds and fruit.

Spicy Bircher Muesli

This Bircher muesli incorporates a grated apple with some complementary spices. This recipe takes ever so slightly longer to make but the results are delicious.

SERVES 2–4

50g porridge oats (gluten-free optional)
50ml apple juice
Pinch of cinnamon
Small pinch of nutmeg
Small pinch of cloves
1 sweet apple, grated
2 tbsp Greek yogurt
1 tsp honey (optional)

1   Mix all the ingredients, except the honey, together with 100ml of water.
2   Leave to soak overnight.
3   Stir and taste. Add honey if not sweet enough. Serve in lunchbox containers.

Protein Yogurt

A while ago a whole range of 'protein' products appeared on our shelves as the world cottoned on to the fact that protein keeps us fuller for longer. Some of these products are not very natural at all and some of the big food players have cashed in on this trend by manufacturing food products that lack nutrients but provide high levels of protein in alarming numbers.

However, there are also products available that are based on real foods and real ingredients. Protein yogurts tend to be such an example. When you look at the label, they should contain simply quark (a cream cheese-like product made in Germany from just one ingredient – milk), yogurt and fruit purée. This home-made version is just as simple and might just save you some money.

SERVES 2

100g Greek yogurt
100g quark
2 tbsp frozen berries
1 tsp honey

1   Mix the ingredients in a bowl and leave in the fridge overnight for the flavours to merge.
2   Serve in 2 containers the following day.

Kefir and Granola

Kefir is like a drinking yogurt. It's a fermented dairy product that has been consumed in eastern Europe and Russia for centuries. As we start to understand more about the role of a healthy digestive system in overall health and wellbeing, so we are introducing more fermented foods into our diets. Kefir is an easy food to introduce into lunches as it's not that different in taste to a drinking yogurt and can be combined with other familiar ingredients for a nutritious yogurt alternative. In this case, the kefir is mixed with some low-sugar granola. Lower sugar granolas are those with less than 5g of sugar per 100g of granola.

SERVES 1–2

120ml kefir
60g low-sugar granola

1 Mix the 2 ingredients in a bowl and leave in the fridge overnight.
2 The following morning, serve the mix in a leakproof lunchbox container or 2.

Dairy-free Chocolate Pot

A rich pot of chocolate that tastes far more decadent than it is.

½ x 400g tin of full-fat coconut milk (make sure you get some of the thick, creamy part as well as the liquid part if the contents of the can have separated)
1 egg yolk
15g maple syrup
Pinch of sea salt
70g chocolate chips

1   Place the coconut milk in a medium saucepan.
2   Whisk in the egg yolk, maple syrup and salt.
3   Heat over a medium heat for 5–10 minutes, stirring constantly.
4   Remove the saucepan from the heat and stir in the chocolate chips until melted.
5   Transfer the mixture to a food processor.
6   Process on high for 40 seconds
7   Place in 2 lunchbox containers.
8   Refrigerate overnight then serve in your lunchbox the following day.

Healthy Chocolate Mousse

The quark in this mousse provides a thick and creamy taste despite being virtually fat-free. It is a great source of protein, making this a filling lunchtime dessert. Younger palates might need some more sweetness. Just add some honey if this is the case.

SERVES 2

90g dark chocolate chips
175g quark
½ tsp cinnamon (optional)
1 tsp honey (optional)

1   Melt the chocolate chips. You can do this in a bowl over a saucepan of simmering water – just don't let the bowl touch the water.
2   Set aside the melted chocolate.
3   In a medium mixing bowl, whisk the quark for a minute or 2 until it becomes light and fluffy.
4   Whisk in the cinnamon, if you like.
5   Whisk in the melted chocolate until the mixture is thick and well-combined.
6   Stir in the honey, if using.
7   Place the mixture in a couple of lunchbox containers and refrigerate overnight.
8   Serve in your lunchbox the next day.

Banana Chia Porridge

Porridge doesn't have to be just for breakfast! This is a portable porridge dish that's ultra-filling and full of goodness. Some like to add a little maple syrup for some extra sweetness.

SERVES 2

30g oats
30g quinoa flakes
20g chia seeds
1 banana, sliced
180ml milk (non-dairy optional)

1   Bring all of the ingredients, plus 260ml of water, to the boil in a medium saucepan and simmer for 5 minutes.
2   Serve with maple syrup, a little more fruit and a little more milk if required in 2 preheated flasks.

Lighter Eton Mess

A favourite dessert for many. The meringues really do bring out the best flavours in the strawberries. This version is made using yogurt rather than cream, a more traditional ingredient. The meringues are distributed evenly throughout the dessert to bring sweetness but not an overpowering sugary taste.

MAKES 2

80g strawberries, washed, stalks removed and quartered
4 mini meringues (about 20g), crumbled
160g thick Greek yogurt

1   Mix all the ingredients together in a medium bowl.
2   Divide the mixture into 2 lunch containers and refrigerate overnight.
3   Serve in your lunchbox.

11 Have Your Cake and Eat It

Have you heard the quote, 'Cake is the answer no matter what the question'? Most people love a bit of cake. For most people, cakes are associated with celebrations and joy. Cakes are brought out at birthdays, weddings, parties, gatherings or, if you're lucky enough to be invited to one, an afternoon tea. Despite its associations with these events, I'd argue that we don't have to reserve cake only for special occasions. In fact, providing we adjust the portion size and the ingredients, we can achieve a healthier, more balanced way of enjoying cake on a more regular basis, even in our lunches.

Healthier alternatives to the main components of cake are readily available. Perhaps for health reasons you prefer to avoid certain ingredients or eat less of them, sugar for example. Where food allergies and intolerances exist, you'll want to know which alternatives you can use instead of common cake ingredients, such as eggs, flour and dairy products. Often when you use healthier alternatives in recipes, the flavour or texture may differ, so it's good to know a few tricks and tips to make sure that your healthier bake is a success.

Fats

Fats are a necessary ingredient in cake making. Why?

Fats keep your cake light (honest!). If you take out the fat and use liquids instead (water, fruit juice, etc.) the cake becomes flat and chewy. It's important to leave the fats in to help protect the protein in the flour. That's why swapping in a low-fat ingredient changes the density.

Fat traps bubbles of air. Many baking recipes have you cream the fat and sugars together as the first step. There's a good reason for that. As you cream these two ingredients together, you add air bubbles. These bubbles help make the cake rise during baking.

Fat improves the moistness of cakes. The fat doesn't evaporate during cooking, nor is it absorbed by other ingredients, unlike liquids.

Which fats to use?

Ideal fats are those that are in a solid state at room temperature – for this reason, butter and coconut oil work really well. By using fats like this you can whip in lots of air bubbles at the start.

Eggs

Egg yolks can be used in place of some of the fat in a cake. They have a binding property and can make cakes richer and denser. They do, of course, also contain some fat.

Egg whites can be whipped into a meringue and gently folded into a cake mixture towards the end of your pre-bake prep to give a light and fluffy texture.

Whether you split the yolk from the white or not it's a good idea to beat eggs well before adding them to a cake mixture.

Eggs allow your cake to rise, too. The proteins unwind and stretch to form a flexible, elastic film that encases air bubbles.

Duck eggs are rich in protein and some who cannot tolerate chickens eggs can in fact tolerate duck eggs. They tend to be larger than chickens eggs. They also lend themselves better to baking, so if you can afford to use duck eggs, it is worth it.

What if you cannot tolerate eggs? There are lots of egg alternatives available for baking. You can replace 1 egg with:

- 2 heaped tbsp arrowroot powder plus 2 tbsp water
- 2 heaped tbsp potato starch powder plus 2 tbsp water
- 1 tbsp ground flaxseeds or chia seeds plus 3 tbsp of warm water
- 3 tbsp fruit purée, e.g. apple purée
- ½ a medium-sized banana, mashed

Sugars

When baking cakes, I recommend reducing the sugar in the recipe you are using by one-third, though not in my recipes, of course, because I have already reduced the sugar content to the right level. You should not notice a discernible difference in flavour and you are doing everyone a healthy favour.

See if you can reduce the sugar even further by adding naturally sweet ingredients, such as carrots, beetroots, apples, pears, berries or bananas. These ingredients can all add sweetness, moistness and fibre to your bake.

If you want to use sugar, then certain types of sugars provide advantages over refined sugar:

Rapadura – This is the most nutrient-dense of the unrefined sugars that you can buy. It is difficult to source, and you may need to buy it online. It's worth it though. You can use this exactly as you would sugar but it has a lower glycaemic index, meaning it releases sugar into the body more slowly once consumed than other sugars. That has distinct health advantages. It also has a lovely caramel flavour.

Coconut sugar – Coconut sugar is evaporated coconut nectar. It is another lower glycaemic option when compared to refined sugar. It has a slightly milder taste than rapadura but is easier to get hold of in mainstream health food stores and even some supermarkets.

Stevia – The fantastic thing about stevia is that it has a glycaemic index of 0. It is a very natural product because it comes from the leaves of the stevia plant. You only need about 1 teaspoon of stevia powder instead of 200g of sugar. This means your cake will have less volume and may be slightly drier, so make sure you reduce the baking tin size and baking temperature by 25 per cent; add an additional egg white or slightly increase the quantity of baking powder/soda; and add fruit purée or yogurt for moistness.

Pure stevia has one downside in that it has a slightly bitter aftertaste. That's not to everyone's liking so manufacturers have started to combine pure stevia with erythritol (a sugar alcohol). Using any sugar alcohol in large quantities can cause digestive discomfort.

Raw honey – You tend to have to buy this from a health food store or online. Raw honey is very easy for our body to digest and has a lower glycaemic index than refined sugar. As it is quite sweet you don't need to use as much. If a recipe calls for 200g of sugar you could use 125g of raw honey, for example. You may need to drop your oven temperature a little and cook the cake for slightly longer as honey can burn more easily than sugar.

Blackstrap molasses – Blackstrap molasses is a byproduct of refined sugar production. It contains vitamins and minerals, such as iron, calcium, magnesium, vitamin B6 and selenium. It provides a fantastically rich taste and tends to be best combined with a little unrefined sugar, such as rapadura or coconut sugar. You can buy this from supermarkets or health food stores. It is not expensive.

Pure maple syrup – This is boiled down from the sap of the maple tree and can be used in the same way as honey. Always use real maple syrup, not maple-flavoured. Like honey, maple syrup can burn, so you may need to lower the temperature of your oven and cook for longer if necessary.

Coconut blossom nectar – This has a mineral-rich flavour like molasses and the sweetness of maple syrup. It also has a lower glycaemic index than sugar and is a great addition to healthier bakes.

Yacon root syrup – Extracted from the roots of the yacon plant, yacon syrup is dark brown in colour and tastes similar to molasses. It is one of the lowest glycaemic sweeteners and also contains higher levels of prebiotic sugars, which make this a particularly health-giving option.

The choice of sugar is yours. The more unrefined and natural sugars retain more nutrients and have a richer flavour, but if you only have refined white sugar or simply standard unrefined sugar in the house, don't let that stop you making the recipe. If you want some of the sugars outlined above, you can always try them at a later date.

Flours

While most baked recipes will call for white wheat flour, there are other options. These are outlined below, with the advantages of each highlighted.

Wholegrain flour – While this will give a denser texture than white flour, the health benefits will be far greater. Wholemeal flour will increase the fibre content and make your cake more filling. It also provides a slightly nutty flavour. I tend to recommend using organic flour or 'ancient grains' (see below) over non-organic wheat flour for health reasons.

Spelt, einkorn and kamut – Opt for spelt or even einkorn or kamut over wheat flour. These are collectively known as 'ancient grains'. They have been grown in a more traditional way with less exposure to herbicides and pesticides. There is some evidence to suggest that the rise in wheat sensitivity among adults and children is due to the use of chemicals in growing wheat just before harvesting to increase yield. Ancient grains tend to have fewer calories than wheat and are higher in protein.

If you want a gluten-free cake, try using naturally gluten-free flours such as buckwheat, brown rice flour, gluten-free oat flour or quinoa flour:

Brown rice flour – This is especially good when combined with other flours, such as buckwheat. You can also make your own by processing brown rice to a powder in a good-quality food processor.

Buckwheat flour – This isn't a grain at all (in fact it is known as a 'pseudo-grain'), which can be confusing because of its name. It's nutrient-dense being a source of minerals, soluble and insoluble fibre as well as antioxidants. Buckwheat flour has a very particular flavour and it is not to everyone's taste, so you can mix it with other flours in a baking recipe. You may find you're fine to use this as the only flour in cakes and bakes so long as you use stronger flavours, such as chocolate, to mask the buckwheat flavour.

Gluten-free oat flour – A great source of fibre, oats can be quite simply made into flour by grinding down whole gluten-free oats. When used in recipes, a little more liquid needs to be added.

Quinoa flour – Quinoa flour is unique in that it has a very high protein content. As with buckwheat, quinoa is not actually a grain but a pseudo-grain. It also has a slight aftertaste, so you may want to blend the flour with other flours and/or use it with stronger flavours.

If you're looking for grain-free and gluten-free bakes, then these flours and starches are useful:

Coconut flour – This flour is made from dried coconut flesh. It is high in fibre, low in carbohydrates and a good source of protein. Recipes using coconut flour will need a lot more liquid and will also require less sugar because coconut has a natural sweetness to it. In baked goods, you generally want to substitute 25g of coconut flour for 130g of grain-based flour. You will also need to increase the number of eggs. In general, for every 115g of coconut flour you use, you will need to use six beaten eggs in your recipe in addition to approximately 250ml of liquid, such as coconut milk.

Tapioca flour – This is an extremely smooth flour that adds a sweetness and chewiness to baking. It can also be used as a thickener. In general, you will use this alongside other grain-free flours in a recipe. An alternative to this is **arrowroot starch**. While neither are especially nutrient-dense they are a useful addition to grain-free bakes and the two can be used interchangeably.

Almond flour – This type of flour is made from ground almonds that have been blanched and their skins removed. It can be used as a 1:1 substitute for wheat flour, but you will need to add more eggs to help bind the flour together as almond flour lacks gluten, and use less butter/coconut oil because nuts contain more fat than wheat.

Green banana flour – This type of flour can replace any plain or wheat flour in a recipe, too. If using in place of wheat flour you'll probably need about 25 per cent less green banana flour than the recipe calls for in wheat flour. It is a form of resistant starch, which means it breaks down into sugars more slowly than other flours and may help balance blood sugar levels.

Black beans – If you are making brownies, try using one cup of puréed black beans instead of 125g of flour. You won't be able to taste the beans, and they give the brownies a delicious fudgy texture.

Happy Baking!

Recipes

Raspberry Tahini Quinoa Bars

This is a moist, fruity and wholesome bar. Remember, quinoa comes in flakes too, which is what this recipe uses – you might otherwise use oats here. Tahini or any other seed or nut butter is used to bind all the ingredients and hold them together.

MAKES 6–8 PORTIONS

145g butter, chopped into cubes, plus extra for greasing
75g coconut sugar or unrefined sugar
1 heaped tbsp of tahini or another seed/nut butter
3 tbsp frozen berries (about 20 frozen berries)
225g quinoa flakes

1 Preheat the oven to 200°C/Fan 180°C/Gas 6.
2 Place the butter and sugar into a medium saucepan.
3 Once melted and combined, stir in the tahini or other seed/nut butter.
4 Stir in the frozen raspberries until they are defrosted and have started to break down.
5 Remove from the heat and stir in the quinoa flakes.
6 Grease 6–8 sections of a 12-hole brownie tin.
7 Fill these with the mixture.
8 Bake for 20 minutes.
9 Take out of the oven and leave to cool before removing them from the tin. Serve in your lunchbox once cooled.

Blueberry and Banana Spelt Bread

This deliciously moist banana and blueberry loaf derives its sweetness from fruit and unrefined sugars. Spelt flour has been chosen in preference to wheat for better digestion, absorption and slower energy release, but you could use wheat flour in place of spelt flour in this recipe if that's what you have or prefer.

MAKES 1 LOAF

125g soft butter, plus extra for greasing
2 large ripe bananas
125ml maple syrup or honey
2 medium eggs
1 tbsp vanilla extract
40ml non-dairy or dairy milk
275g wholegrain spelt flour
1 tsp bicarbonate of soda
½ tsp baking powder
½ tsp salt
150g blueberries

1   Preheat the oven to 200°C/Fan 180°C/Gas 6.
2   Grease and line a 2lb loaf tin with greaseproof paper.
3   Mash the bananas with the back of a fork. Leave to one side.
4   Mix the butter, maple syrup or honey, eggs, vanilla and milk together until combined.
5   In a separate bowl, combine the flour, bicarbonate of soda, baking powder and salt.
6   Add the banana and the 'wet' ingredients (butter, maple syrup or honey, eggs, etc.) and stir to combine completely.
7   Add 110g of the blueberries to the mixture and fold them in gently.
8   Pour the mix into the greased loaf tin and scatter the remaining 40g of berries over the top.
9   Bake for approximately 50 minutes. Check that it is cooked through by inserting a cocktail stick into the loaf. If it comes out clean the loaf is cooked. Remove from the oven.
10 Leave to cool then remove from the pan and slice for lunches.

Raspberry Chia Flapjacks

This is a moist, fruity and fibre-rich flapjack. The raspberries bring
a delicious tartness that contrasts so well with the wholesome
combination of oats, butter or coconut oil and chia seeds.

MAKES 8 PORTIONS

55g chia seeds
150g oats
100g butter or coconut oil
75g honey
150g frozen raspberries, left to thaw for at least 3 hours then mulched
with the back of a fork
½ tsp butter or coconut oil, for greasing

1   Preheat the oven to 200°C/Fan 180°C/Gas 6.
2   Grind the chia seeds in a food processor to form a powder. Stir
    in the oats. Melt the butter or oil and the honey in a saucepan
    then stir this into the chia/oat mix.
3   Stir in the raspberries. Grease 8 sections of a 12-hole brownie
    tin. Pour the mixture in. Bake for 20 minutes until cooked
    through.
4   Remove then leave to cool before serving in your lunchbox.

Green Banana Flour and Chocolate Chip Drop Scones

Green banana flour may sound a bit quirky, but this flour is a useful one to know about, especially if you are looking for something with slower-release carbohydrates and a sweet treat that will keep you fuller for longer than other options. These little drop scones are a great lunchbox filler.

MAKES ABOUT 10 DROP SCONES

110g green banana flour
½ tsp bicarbonate of soda
2 eggs or 2 flax eggs (2 tbsp ground flaxseeds soaked in 6 tbsp warm water for 10 minutes)
½ tsp vanilla extract
1 tsp apple cider vinegar
180ml milk (non-dairy optional)
60g dark chocolate chips
1 tsp avocado or olive oil

1   In a medium-sized bowl, stir together the banana flour and bicarbonate of soda.
2   In another bowl mix the eggs, vanilla and cider vinegar together with the milk.
3   Combine the flour mixture with the wet ingredients – eggs, vanilla, vinegar and milk – then gently fold in the chocolate chips.
4   Heat the oil in a pan. Add spoonfuls of the batter to the hot oil. Flip each drop scone after 1–2 minutes and cook them on the other side. Remove them from the pan.
5   Cool then serve in your lunchbox.

Chocolate-covered German Biscuits

At Christmas time my family like to eat something called 'Lebkuchen' biscuits from Germany. They are simply the taste of Christmas. A wonderful celebration of the flavours of this time in a soft and mildly spicy biscuit. This is our home-made version.

MAKES ABOUT 30 BISCUITS

100g butter, softened
1 egg
60g honey or coconut nectar
25g maple syrup
300g ground almonds
1½ tsp ground ginger
½ tsp allspice
½ tsp ground cinnamon
1 tsp bicarbonate of soda
Pinch of salt
4 tbsp coconut flour, plus extra for rolling
200g dark chocolate

1   Preheat the oven to 190°C/Fan 170°C/Gas 5.
2   Combine the butter, egg, honey and maple syrup in a bowl.
3   In a separate bowl, combine the ground almonds, spices, bicarbonate of soda and salt.
4   Combine the wet ingredients with the spice mixture. Add in 4 tablespoons of coconut flour and stir well.
5   Using the extra coconut flour, roll the dough out to a 1cm thickness.
6   Cut shapes from the rolled-out dough. Place on a baking sheet lined with greaseproof paper (you will need 2 or 3 large baking sheets).
7   Bake for 13 minutes or until golden brown.
8   Remove, and leave to cool.
9   Melt the chocolate in a bowl over simmering water.
10 Dip the cooled biscuits in, covering the whole biscuit.
11 Leave to cool on a non-stick silicone sheet.

Half-and-half Chickpea Cookies – Raisin or Chocolate

These cookies combine cooked chickpeas with slower energy-release spelt flour and a little sweetness from raisins and chocolate chips. The reason there's half raisin and half chocolate is that people seem to fall into two camps when it comes to cookies: chocolate chip lovers or raisin lovers. This way everybody is happy.

MAKES 16–20 COOKIES

400g cooked chickpeas (tinned is fine but you want 400g drained weight, so a 400g tin is insufficient as this yields less than 300g of chickpeas)

110g wholegrain spelt flour

1 tsp baking powder

75g melted butter

2 tbsp coconut milk

½ tsp vanilla extract

½ tsp ground cinnamon

1–2 tbsp honey

70g chocolate chips

70g raisins

1   Preheat the oven to 200°C/Fan 180°C/Gas 6.
2   In a food processor, whizz the cooked chickpeas to as fine a paste as possible.
3   Add the flour and baking powder and process again.
4   Stir in the melted butter, milk, vanilla, cinnamon and honey. Bring together into a big ball of dough then tear into 2 halves.
5   Add the chocolate chips to one half.
6   Add the raisins to the other half.
7   Roll each dough into table-tennis-sized balls.
8   Place the balls on to baking trays lines with parchment. Flatten the cookies with your fingers. You should be able to make between 8–10 of each type.
9   Bake for 15–20 minutes until golden brown on top. Remove the cookies from the oven and put them on a cooling rack.
10 Place in your lunchbox once cool.

Coconut Apple Slices

These moist slices are suited to those who want a healthier, grain-free cake. Coconut flour requires more eggs and more moisture than wheat flour. The moisture in this case comes from apple purée, which also provides a comforting sweetness and a taste of autumn.

MAKE 9 PORTIONS

45g melted coconut oil, melted but not hot, plus extra for greasing
270g apple purée
30g maple syrup
1 tsp vanilla extract
5 medium eggs, beaten
85g coconut flour
1½ tsp ground cinnamon
1 tsp bicarbonate of soda

1   Preheat the oven to 200°C/Fan 180°C/Gas 6.
2   Grease 9 sections of a 12-hole brownie tin with coconut oil.
3   In a bowl, mix the coconut oil, apple purée, maple syrup, vanilla extract and eggs together.
4   In another bowl, mix the flour, cinnamon and bicarbonate of soda together.
5   Combine the wet and the dry ingredients and stir well, then leave them to sit for 5 minutes. During this time, the batter will thicken but remain airy.
6   Place the mixture evenly into the 9 sections in the tin.
7   Bake for 20 minutes. Make sure they are cooked all the way through by inserting a cocktail stick into the centre and checking it comes out clean. Leave to cool.
8   Serve with a little yogurt, coconut cream or cream.

Oat-based Chocolate Chip Cookies

If you're a fan of peanut butter cookies, then you'll like these moist, chewy almond-butter-based cookies made with oats and chocolate chips.

MAKES 8 BISCUITS

150g crunchy almond nut butter
40g honey
90g rolled oats (gluten-free optional)
½ tsp bicarbonate of soda
A pinch of salt
1 large egg
60g dark chocolate chips

1 Preheat the oven to 200°C/Fan 180°C/Gas 6.
2 Melt the nut butter and honey in a small saucepan over a low heat. As soon as they have mixed together, remove the pan from the heat.
3 In a medium-sized bowl, mix the oats, bicarbonate of soda and salt together, then combine with the nut butter and honey mix. Then gradually stir in the egg.
4 Add the chocolate chips and stir until evenly distributed.
5 Using your hands, mould the mixture into about 8 biscuits and place on to a lined baking sheet.
6 Bake for 12–14 minutes until firm to the touch. Cool well then pack into lunchboxes.

Gluten-free Chocolate Chip Cookies

This tastes just like a chocolate chip cookie from one of the major coffee chains, according to my teenager. That's high commendation indeed. The reality is that this recipe is gluten-free, wholegrain and way lower in sugar than the branded cookie so there are a multitude of pluses.

MAKES 10 COOKIES

130g butter, softened, plus extra for greasing
180g buckwheat flour
1 tsp baking powder
95g coconut blossom nectar or honey
1 tsp vanilla extract
1 egg or 1 flax egg (1 tbsp ground flaxseeds left to soak in 3 tbsp warm water for 10 minutes)
60g dark chocolate chips
30g chopped nuts

1   Preheat the oven to 180°C/Fan 160°C/Gas 5.
2   Grease 2 large baking trays.
3   Mix the flour and baking powder together in a bowl.
4   In another bowl, beat together the butter and coconut blossom nectar or honey. Add the vanilla and egg or flax egg to this.
5   Stir in the chocolate chips and nuts.
6   Using your hands, roll the dough into 10 equal-sized balls.
7   Place the balls on 2 baking trays leaving 3cm or so between each cookie.
8   Bake for 15–20 minutes or until golden brown on the top.
9   Cool on a cooling rack.
10 Place in your lunchbox once cool.

Chocolate Protein Brownie Balls

These protein brownies are ideal for sporty types, and as they're raw there's no need to bake them. They combine fruity and sweet dates with protein in the form of powder and nuts or seeds with cocoa or cacao for antioxidants.

MAKES 10 BALLS

40g walnuts (for a nut-free version use sunflower or pumpkin seeds)
A pinch of salt
130g whole pitted dates
1 heaped tbsp of plant-based protein powder (hemp, pea or rice)
½ tsp vanilla extract
15g pure cocoa or cacao powder

1   In a food processor, grind the walnuts or seeds with the pinch of salt.
2   Add the dates and protein powder to the nuts or seeds and blend.
3   Add the vanilla and cocoa powder. Blend again.
4   The mixture should stick together nicely when pinched.
5   Roll into equal-sized balls (a little smaller than a golf ball).
6   Place in the fridge and allow to cool, ideally for 2 hours, before packing into a lunchbox. These need to be kept cool in order to keep their shape.

Chocolate Orange Flapjacks

Chocolate and orange are a delightful flavour combination, but rarely do you see them combined in a flapjack. The two flavours just work in this moist and chocolaty treat.

MAKES 6–8 PORTIONS

120g butter, plus extra for greasing
50g unrefined or coconut sugar
225g oats or gluten-free oats
50g dark chocolate chips, plus 20g to decorate
½ tsp vanilla extract
6 drops of food-grade orange oil
1 egg or 1 flax egg (1 tbsp ground flaxseeds left to soak in 3 tbsp warm water for 10 minutes)

1   Preheat the oven to 200°C/Fan 180°C/Gas 6.
2   Melt the butter and sugar in a medium saucepan.
3   Stir in the oats, dark chocolate chips (except the 20g for decoration), vanilla and orange oil.
4   Then stir in the egg or flax egg.
5   Grease a shallow square baking tin of about 20 x 20cm or 6–8 sections of a 12-hole brownie tin. Fill the tin or sections with the mixture, but not quite to the top.
6   Decorate the top with the extra chocolate chips.
7   Bake in the oven for 20 minutes.
8   Remove the tin from the oven. If using a square tin, cut into pieces and leave to cool before removing the flapjacks from the tin. If using a brownie tin, allow to cool before removing the flapjacks.

Apple Flapjacks

The apple and honey provide the sweetness in this seedy flapjack.
Combined with a touch of aromatic cloves, these flapjacks are so
delicious and are a real lunchbox treat.

MAKES 8–10 PORTIONS

1 large or 2 small sweet apples, plus an extra ½ large apple or 1 small
apple, thinly sliced
250g oats or gluten-free oats
¼ tsp ground cloves
2 tbsp pumpkin seeds
2 tbsp sunflower seeds
95g butter
3 tbsp honey

1   Preheat the oven to 200°C/Fan 180°C/Gas 6.
2   Grease and line a 20cm-by-20cm baking tin with greaseproof
    paper.
3   Pop the large apple or 2 small apples into your food processor to
    grate, or grate by hand.
4   Add the oats, cloves and seeds to the apples and mix together.
5   Meanwhile, melt the butter and honey in a saucepan.
6   Pour the melted butter and honey into the oat mix and stir until
    all combined.
7   Pour the mixture out on to a baking tray lined with greaseproof
    paper.
8   Top with the thinly sliced apple evenly spaced.
9   Bake for 20 minutes or until golden brown.
10 Score into pieces once out of the oven but allow to cool before
    removing individual portions from the tray.

Raspberry Muffins

A simple, fruity muffin made with low-sugar fruit and wholegrain flour, which is less likely to harm energy levels than a biscuit, cake or cereal bar.

MAKES 12

250g wholegrain spelt flour
60g coconut, rapadura or unrefined sugar
1 tbsp baking powder
125ml milk
75g melted butter, plus extra for greasing
1 large egg
170g fresh raspberries

1   Preheat the oven to 200°C/Fan 180°C/Gas 6.
2   Grease a 12-hole muffin tin.
3   Mix together the dry ingredients.
4   Mix together the wet ingredients, except the raspberries.
5   Put the wet and dry ingredients together and stir until just combined.
6   Fold in the raspberries.
7   Place the mixture into your muffin tray.
8   Bake for 20–25 minutes or until a cocktail stick inserted into the muffin comes out clean.

Sugar-free Oat Cookies

These cookies are just great for lunchboxes. As they are egg-, dairy- and nut-free they will suit those with allergies to any of those groups. They're full of fibre and they taste delicious. They are also incredibly easy to make.

MAKES 12 COOKIES

Coconut oil, for greasing
90g rolled oats
50g ground sunflower seeds or pumpkin seeds (use a food processor to grind them into a powder/flour)
100g desiccated coconut (unsweetened)
¼ tsp cinnamon
¼ tsp nutmeg
½ tsp baking powder
3 medium-sized ripe bananas, peeled
½ tsp vanilla extract
75g coconut oil, melted
A good handful of any of the following: unsulphured dried apricots cut into very small pieces, raisins, or cranberries.

1   Preheat the oven to 200°C/Fan 180°C/Gas 6.
2   Grease 2 baking sheets with some coconut oil.
3   Combine the oats, ground seeds, desiccated coconut, cinnamon, nutmeg and baking powder in a bowl.
4   In a second bowl, mash together the bananas, vanilla extract and coconut oil.
5   Combine the wet and dry ingredients in the food processor and add the handful of dried fruit. Do not process, just mix at this stage to keep the latest ingredients intact.
6   Using your hands, make the dough into about 12 balls then flatten them into cookies and place them on to the baking trays.
7   Bake for about 20 minutes or until golden brown.
8   Transfer to a cooling rack when they are cool enough to handle.

Quinoa Banana Maple Slice

This banana maple slice is made with just five ingredients and with very few steps. As with other quinoa flake recipes, oats and quinoa flakes can be used interchangeably. The banana and maple flavours make this taste deliciously sweet for those with a sweeter tooth.

MAKES ABOUT 7 PORTIONS

100g butter, cubed, plus extra for greasing
75g maple syrup
2 ripe bananas, mashed
1 tsp vanilla extract
240g quinoa flakes

1 Preheat the oven to 200°C/Fan 180°C/Gas 6.
2 Grease 7 sections of a 12-hole brownie tin or more if using a muffin tin.
3 Melt the butter and maple syrup together in a medium-sized saucepan.
4 Add the mashed banana and the vanilla extract.
5 Stir in the quinoa flakes.
6 Place the mixture into the sections or holes.
7 Bake for 20–25 minutes until golden brown on top.
8 Leave to cool before removing from the tin.

Gluten-free Banana Bread

Banana bread is a favourite for lots of people, and because bananas are naturally high in sugar you won't add a lot of sugar to this moist, sumptuous cake. It's made gluten-free, using a home-made gluten-free flour mix (buckwheat, brown rice flour, arrowroot, ground flaxseeds).

MAKES 1 LOAF

80g buckwheat flour
50g brown rice flour
25g tapioca starch or arrowroot powder starch
20g ground flaxseeds
1 tsp bicarbonate of soda
A pinch of salt
75g coconut sugar or rapadura
4 bananas, mashed
1 egg or 1 flax egg (1 tbsp ground flaxseeds left to soak in 3 tbsp warm water for 10 minutes)
75g butter, softened, plus extra for greasing
1 tsp vanilla extract

1   Preheat the oven to 180°C/Fan 160°C/Gas 4.
2   Grease and line a 2lb loaf tin.
3   In a large bowl, mix together the dry ingredients – flours, tapioca/arrowroot, bicarbonate of soda, salt and sugar.
4   In a separate bowl, mix together the wet ingredients – bananas, egg/flax egg, butter and vanilla.
5   Add the wet ingredients to the dry ingredients. Stir to combine.
6   Pour the batter into your loaf tin.
7   Bake for about 1 hour. Check that it is cooked completely by inserting a cocktail stick. If clean when removed, the cake is cooked.
8   Take out of the oven and leave to cool before removing from the tin.

12 Drinks for Concentration

Dehydration

It is far easier than one might think to become dehydrated. In a survey of 3,003 Americans, 75 per cent were found to be chronically dehydrated. While this might come as a surprise, it is common for people to become dehydrated not only because they don't drink enough but also because they eat too much sodium or consume too many caffeinated drinks, which are diuretics, i.e. they speed up the rate at which we lose liquid.

Signs of dehydration include:

- Little or no urine
- Urine that is darker than usual. It should be the colour of straw or lighter
- Dry mouth
- Sleepiness or fatigue
- Extreme thirst
- Headache
- Confusion
- Dizziness or light-headedness
- No tears when crying

If your urine is usually colourless or light yellow, you are well hydrated. If your urine is a dark yellow or amber colour, you may be dehydrated.

Though water is the number-one choice of fluid, fruit and vegetable juices, milk and herbal teas add to the amount of water you get each day. Even caffeinated drinks such as coffee and tea can contribute to your daily water intake as long as they are consumed in moderation. A moderate amount of caffeine – 200–300mg – is not harmful for most people, but caffeinated drinks are diuretics so this should be considered in your overall hydration plan.

Water can also be found in fruit and vegetables – for example, in watermelon, celery, cucumber, tomatoes and lettuce – and in soups and broths. These too count towards your daily water intake.

If staying hydrated is difficult for you, overleaf are some tips that can help:

- Keep a bottle of water with you during the day. To reduce your costs, carry a reusable water bottle and fill it with filtered tap water.
- If you don't like the taste of water, try adding a slice of lemon or lime to your drink.
- Drink water before, during and after a workout.
- When you're feeling hungry, drink water. Thirst is often confused with hunger. True hunger will not be satisfied by drinking water.
- If you have trouble remembering to drink water, drink on a schedule. For example, drink water when you wake up, when your first get to work, during a break or meeting and when you go to bed. Or drink a small glass of water at the beginning of each hour.
- Don't wait until you notice symptoms of dehydration to take action. Actively prevent dehydration by drinking plenty of water.

Water makes up more than half of your body weight. You lose water each day when you go to the loo, sweat and even when you breathe. This has to be replaced.

Lunchtime is an opportunity, as is any other meal, for both hydration and optimising nutrient intake. The drink recipes that follow provide both water/liquid and natural ingredients that are designed for optimal nutritional intake.

If you want to build a healthy smoothie, then a green smoothie is a really simple and healthy one to try. It's also really easy to make your own version by following some simple steps:

Green Smoothies
Step 1: Choose a liquid base – milk, almond milk, coconut milk, coconut water, rice milk, water.
Step 2: Add your greens – spinach, kale or lettuce.
Step 3: Add your fruit – apple, banana, mango, berries, citrus.
Step 4: Add your 'BOOSTER' – ginger, avocado, chia seeds, flaxseeds, coconut oil, cinnamon, nut butter.

If you're not a green smoothie fan, then there are plenty of other fruit- and vegetable-based drinks that you can try.

Ideal Ingredients for Smoothies

Smoothies are not only an opportunity to include vegetables or fruit in your lunchbox in the form of a drink, nor are they only a source of hydration: they can also provide an opportunity to increase the consumption of filling proteins.

Proteins

Ideal proteins to include in a smoothie are: quark (which is actually a cheese with a thick yogurt-like consistency), yogurt, plant-based protein powders, chia seeds, flaxseeds, nut butters, seed butters, seeds, nuts, oats, oat flour, quinoa flakes.

The liquid base for a smoothie is an important consideration and must match the other ingredients in terms of complementary flavours.

Liquids

The range of liquids you could put in a smoothie is vast but can include fruit juices, vegetable juices, dairy milk, non-dairy milk, coconut water, coconut milk, and even water.

Frozen Ingredients

Smoothies must be served and consumed at the right temperature for optimal enjoyment. It is recommended that you include at least one frozen ingredient, such as berries, spinach, banana, avocado or ice cubes, in your smoothie as this not only improves texture but also palatability as a result of keeping the smoothie cooler for longer.

Recipes

The following recipes for lunchbox drinks are all simple and quick to make. The idea is to pack taste and nutrients into each drink whilst also providing hydration.

Berry Banana 'Milk' Shake

This is an ideal drink on a hot day as coconut water is known to be particularly efficient at replacing electrolytes. You'll see that there is no actual milk in this shake, but the combination of fruit, coconut water and yogurt does create a milky texture.

SERVES 2

100g frozen blueberries
1 small ripe banana
1 tbsp chia seeds
110g Greek yogurt
220ml coconut water

1   Combine all the ingredients in a food processor.
2   Keep cold until ready to drink.

Berry Smoothie

A simple combination of berries with milk and yogurt and a touch
of natural sweetness make up this delicious fruit smoothie.

SERVES 1

2 tbsp frozen blueberries
2 tbsp frozen raspberries
100ml rice milk
100g Greek yogurt
¼ tsp raw honey

1   Combine all the ingredients in a food processor.
2   Keep cold until ready to drink.

Mango Smoothie

This juicy orange-coloured smoothie is full of complementary flavours.

1 medium mango, flesh only
Juice of 1 orange
Juice of ½ lemon
240ml milk

1   Process the ingredients together in a food processor.
2   Keep cold until ready to drink.

Watermelon Froth

An immensely refreshing taste of the tropics, combining the
rehydrating properties of watermelon with creamy coconut milk
and flakes.

SERVES 2

250g watermelon chunks
45ml coconut milk from a carton or can
1 tbsp coconut flakes
1/8 tsp vanilla extract
2 ice cubes

1   Place all ingredients in a food processor and process until
    smooth.
2   Keep cold until ready to drink.

Strawberry Banana Milkshake

A classic fruit combination and one most people of all ages will enjoy immensely.

SERVES 2

1 banana, cut into pieces
10 strawberries
250ml dairy or non-dairy milk

1   Place the banana pieces in a plastic bag and freeze for at least an hour.
2   In a food processor, process all the ingredients together until the strawberries are broken and the milkshake is frothy and thick.
3   Keep cold until ready to drink.

Fruity Kefir Shake

Kefir is a probiotic yogurt drink that has been consumed in eastern Europe and Russia for centuries. It's known for its health-boosting properties and we are now starting to understand why, as our knowledge about the role friendly bacteria plays increases.

SERVES 2

250ml kefir
100g frozen fruit
100g fresh fruit
A squeeze of yacon syrup (a prebiotic syrup) or raw honey (optional)

1   Mix the ingredients together in a food processor.
2   Keep cold until ready to drink.

Chocolate Chia Milk

A healthier take on chocolate milkshake. Full of nutrients, from the antioxidant-rich cacao to the omega 3-rich chia seeds.

400ml dairy or non-dairy milk
150g Greek or non-dairy (coconut) yogurt
1 frozen banana
1 tbsp cocoa/cacao powder
2 tbsp chia seeds
2 tsp maple syrup or raw honey

1   Mix the ingredients together in a food processor.
2   Keep cold until ready to drink.

Blueberry, Banana
and Avocado Smoothie

This creamy berry smoothie surprises many with its 'shock'
ingredient – the avocado. As with other smoothies containing this
ingredient, it is there for creaminess and not flavour.

SERVES 2

180g frozen blueberries
1 ripe banana
1 ripe avocado
3 ice cubes

1   Place all the ingredients into a food processor with 250ml of
    water and process until smooth.
2   Keep cold until ready to drink.

Green Smoothie

Green smoothies have been a bit of a thing for some time. They are so simple to create and to my mind a great way to 'eat your greens' without actually having to eat them.

SERVES 2

Handful of baby spinach
250ml coconut water
1 apple
1 ripe pear
½ ripe avocado, sliced
Juice of ½ lime
2 ice cubes

1 Place all the ingredients into a food processor and process until smooth.
2 Keep cold until ready to drink.

Cucumber Water

This simple combination is refreshing and essentially little more than flavoured water.

SERVES 2

3 ice cubes
3 thin slices of cucumber, created using a vegetable peeler down the side of a cucumber
500ml water

1 Simply add the ice and cucumber to the water in an insulated bottle.
2 Take to school or work and sip on it throughout the day.
3 Other recommended additions to the water: lime or lemon juice, some mint leaves.

Mango Yogurt Drink

This sweet, creamy mango drink is surprisingly filling.

SERVES 1

1 very ripe mango, peeled and roughly chopped
3 tbsps full-fat Greek-style natural yogurt
150ml dairy or non-dairy milk

1   Blitz the 3 ingredients in a food processor.
2   Keep cold until ready to drink.

Carrot and Mango Smoothie

Carrot and mango combine really well in this deliciously
refreshing orange smoothie.

<u>SERVES 2</u>

200ml carrot juice
1 whole frozen mango, cubed before freezing
3 ice cubes

1   Process the ingredients in a food processor until smooth.
2   Keep cold until ready to drink.

Apple and Beetroot Smoothie

Beetroot is jam-packed full of antioxidants. The bright colours of this smoothie should be a reminder that the brighter the better when it comes to health benefits.

200ml apple juice
1 whole cooked beetroot
75g frozen blueberries
2 tbsp Greek yogurt
A squeeze of lemon juice

1 Process the ingredients in a food processor until smooth.
2 Keep cold until ready to drink.

13 Allergies, Money, the Environment and Top Tips for Kids

Lunchbox Without Allergens

The Rise of Food Allergies and Intolerances

Allergies and intolerances to foods and ingredients are increasingly common. The good news is that if you or your family suffer from an allergy or intolerance, making your own lunches at home to take to work or school means you are in control of exactly what goes into the meal and you can ensure there is no cross-contamination from allergenic ingredients.

However, from a nutritional standpoint simply avoiding the allergens may not lead to the most nutritious lunches. When one or more food groups are avoided it is all too easy to pack lunches devoid of certain nutrients.

Food Allergy

It helps to be aware of the nutrients that some of the most common allergens provide to be able to identify what other foods could provide these nutrients in the lunchbox. The nutrients provided by the foods most commonly causing allergic reactions are:

Dairy	Egg	Soy	Wheat	Peanuts
Vitamin A	Vitamin B12	Vitamin B1	Vitamin B1	Vitamin E
Vitamin D	Vitamin B2	Vitamin B2	Vitamin B2	Niacin
Riboflavin	Vitamin B5	Vitamin B6	Vitamin B3	Magnesium
Pantothenic acid	Biotin	Folate	Iron	Manganese
Vitamin B12	Selenium	Calcium	Folate (if fortified)	Chromium
Calcium		Phosphorous		
Phosphorous		Magnesium		
		Iron		
		Zinc		

If one or more of these foods are avoided for allergy reasons, then the nutrients they might otherwise have provided can be gained by eating other food sources in your lunch.

Note: In brackets you'll find the common allergens that are also sources of these nutrients, as not every allergen affects every person.

Vitamin A	Beans, pumpkin seeds (eggs, dairy, cod liver oil)
Vitamin D	Tinned oily fish (dairy, eggs)
Vitamin B1	Brown rice, meat, non-gluten wholegrains (eggs, nuts, gluten-containing wholegrains, soy)
Vitamin B2	Chicken, turkey, non-gluten wholegrains (eggs, gluten-containing wholegrains, dairy, soy)
Vitamin B3	Potatoes, red meat, fish (non-gluten wholegrains, eggs, nuts, dairy)
Vitamin B5	Beans, peas, lentils, vegetables, mushrooms, non-gluten wholegrains (eggs, gluten-containing wholegrains)
Vitamin B6	Chicken, turkey, carrots, sunflower seeds, peas (eggs, walnuts, soy)
Biotin	Chicken, turkey, non-gluten wholegrains (eggs, gluten-containing wholegrains)
Vitamin E	Green leafy vegetables, avocados, seeds, lentils, peas, beans, non-gluten wholegrains (eggs, gluten-containing wholegrains, nuts)
Selenium	Dark green vegetables, mushrooms, onions, garlic, non-gluten wholegrains (dairy, gluten-containing wholegrains)
Calcium	Dark green leafy vegetables, seeds, root vegetables, canned fish, blackstrap molasses (dairy, nuts, soy)
Magnesium	Dark green leafy vegetables, beans, lentils, peas, dried fruit, garlic, fish, seeds, non-gluten wholegrains (nuts, gluten-containing wholegrains, soy)
Manganese	Dark green leafy vegetables, fruit, fish, root vegetables, non-gluten wholegrains (eggs, nuts, gluten-containing wholegrains)
Iron	Red meat, fish, cacao, green leafy vegetables, lentils, peas, seeds, non-gluten wholegrains, blackstrap molasses (eggs, nuts, gluten-containing wholegrains)
Chromium	Root vegetables, fruit, chicken, turkey, non-gluten wholegrains (eggs, gluten-containing wholegrains, dairy)

This shows that it is entirely feasible to produce a nutritionally balanced lunchbox that is free from the main allergens. It does require some thought and planning and certainly using the Lunchbox Bingo template can help with this. The following plan shows how to create a one-week plan for lunches free from the main allergens while being nutritionally balanced.

Weekly Menu Plan – Free from allergens

MONDAY

	Carbohydrate	Protein	Calcium	Fruit	Vegetable	Drink
Free-from pasta with nut-free pesto and torn cooked chicken	✓	✓	✓			
Watermelon cubes, cucumber cubes and finely chopped mint				✓	✓	
Bottle of water						✓

TUESDAY

	Carbohydrate	Protein	Calcium	Fruit	Vegetable	Drink
Mashed roasted butternut squash and sweetcorn	✓				✓	
Corn tortillas – lightly salted	✓					
Roasted chicken strips and carrot batons, roasted in olive oil		✓			✓	
Dried figs with pumpkin seeds			✓	✓		
Mango lassi – (combine a whole mango, vanilla pod, small tin of coconut cream and lots of ice) in a food processor				✓		✓

WEDNESDAY

	Carbohydrate	Protein	Calcium	Fruit	Vegetable	Drink
Roasted butternut squash, salad leaves, rolled slices of cold roast beef	✓	✓			✓	
Vegetable crisps	✓				✓	
Roasted sunflower seeds		✓	✓			
Fruit smoothie carton				✓		✓

THURSDAY

	Carbohydrate	Protein	Calcium	Fruit	Vegetable	Drink
Tahini-free hummus with broccoli trees			✓		✓	
Free-from pasta with chopped sliced turkey breast, sweetcorn and dressing (olive oil and lemon with salt and pepper)	✓	✓			✓	
Blueberries with orange slices				✓		
Bottle of water						✓

FRIDAY

	Carbohydrate	Protein	Calcium	Fruit	Vegetable	Drink
Wholegrain rice cakes with sunflower seed butter and raisins	✓	✓	✓	✓		
Little gem lettuce wraps – choice of filling i.e. turkey, chicken and pepper strips with thinly sliced cucumber		✓			✓	
Mango hedgehog – half mango cheek served like a hedgehog				✓		
Carton of fortified non-dairy milk			✓			✓

Food Intolerances

Where food intolerances are concerned, there tends to be three main areas to focus on:

- Lactose or dairy intolerance
- Non-coeliac gluten sensitivity and coeliac disease
- Egg intolerance

Let's look at each in terms of packing nutritionally balanced lunches.

Lactose-free Products

There are now many products on the market that market themselves with the name 'Lactose-free'. These include cheeses, milks and yogurts. They can be incredibly useful for those who suffer from lactose intolerance as they contain most of the nutrients of their non-lactose-free alternatives but lack the lactose that causes problems for some.

However, if you prefer organic dairy products you may struggle to find products that are both organic and lactose-free. This is slowly changing as more organic lactose-free products creep on to the market. If you do prefer organic and are lactose-free, then you might be better off opting to omit dairy products that contain lactose from your diet.

Low-lactose Products

If you struggle with digesting too much lactose and therefore seek lower-lactose products, then the following are naturally lower in lactose:

- Butter and ghee
- Lower lactose cheeses:
  - Cheese with trace levels (less than 0.5g of lactose): aged cheeses, such as Cheddar, pecorino, gouda, feta and Parmesan, as most of the lactose is drained off with the whey. The small amount that remains in the curd is changed to lactic acid during ripening (ageing) of the cheese.
  - Cheese with low levels (less than 5g of lactose): non-aged cheeses, such as mozzarella, cream cheese and ricotta. Only part of the lactose that remains in the curd has a chance to convert to lactic acid.

— Cottage cheese should be lower in lactose; however, some brands add milk or cream to the curd. Therefore, look for brands that make pure cottage cheese if you can handle lower-lactose cheeses.

- Probiotic yogurt: because most yogurts contain live bacteria that can help break down lactose, so you don't have as much to digest yourself.
- Kefir: for the same reason as above.

Dairy (i.e. not just lactose)

If you are unable to tolerate dairy produce, then the following recommendations will be useful:

- Use coconut oil, olive oil or seed oils in place of butter. You can freeze both olive oil and seed oils to make it stiffer, like butter, for spreading.
- When baking you can use coconut oil, avocado oil or olive oil in place of butter.
- As a yogurt alternative there are a range of coconut-milk-based and even almond-milk-based yogurts suitable for lunches.
- For adding alternatives to cream to sauces and soups there are a range of dairy-free alternatives made from gluten-free oats or coconut milk/cream.

Eggs

While there are plenty of commercial egg-free alternatives to normally egg-based foods on the market, not all are healthy, nutritionally balanced, real foods. Some brands of egg-free mayonnaise contain fifteen or so ingredients, including thickening agents and sweeteners or sugars, and most contain soy, which is also a common allergen.

Alternatives for dressings and binding sandwich fillings are oils, vinegars, coconut yogurt or a combination of these.

If you are looking for alternatives to eggs when baking:

Ground flax seeds	Chia seeds	Arrowroot powder	Ripe banana	Apple purée
1 tbsp mixed with 3 tbsp warm water	1 tbsp mixed with 3 tbsp warm water	2 tbsp mixed with 2 tbsp water	½ a banana, mashed	65g

Gluten

There are many real-food alternatives to gluten-containing grains. These alternatives include what are known as pseudo-grains, such as buckwheat (not related to wheat) and quinoa, but also legume-based flours, nut flours and non-gluten containing grains.

Non-gluten grain or pseudo grain	How it can be used or eaten
Quinoa	Flakes (can be used like oats), flour, 'grains' (can be used to make porridge and also in place of couscous or bulgur wheat), puffed as a cereal, crackers
Rice	Grain, flakes, flour, puffed, rice cakes, crackers, breads
Buckwheat	Groats (like wholegrains), flour (for use in cakes and pancakes), breads, crispbreads
Millet	Flour, crispbreads, pasta
Chickpeas	Pasta, gram flour (used for pancakes), roasted (as a snack)
Yellow peas	Flour (used in pancakes), roasted (as a snack)
Chestnut	Flour (used in pancakes)
Coconut	Flour (used in baking)
Corn	Flour, polenta (used to make side dishes or snacks), tortillas, popcorn, nachos, crispbreads
Green banana (dried	Flour (for use in cakes and pancakes)

Healthy, nutritionally balanced lunches are perfectly achievable for those with food allergies and intolerances. Making your own lunch to take from home to work or school provides you with the opportunity to get it right, just for you. Real-food alternatives to allergenic foods or ingredients are going to be the best choice, but failing that, choose products with the most recognisable ingredients and the least added ingredients.

Save Money

How Real Food Lunches Can Save Money and the Environment

As supermarkets, food shops and take-away chains have done their best to make the process of buying and eating lunch on the go more convenient, they have done so at a price that suits neither our pocket nor the environment. Bagged portions of fruit, individually wrapped cheeses and bags of crisps are all easy to buy and easy to eat, but they cost us more than if we were to buy a large pack and divide it into portions to be eaten throughout the whole week and maybe into the next week too.

Buy large, serve small

It benefits both you and the environment to buy larger-sized portions and to divide them up into individual portions of certain packed lunch foods. The following are in most cases cheaper when bought in larger sizes and divided up:

- Cheese
- Yogurt
- Crackers
- Healthier crisps
- Vegetables
- Fruit
- Dried fruit
- Dips including hummus, tzatziki, raita, guacamole, salsa
- Olives

In order to understand just how much money this approach could be saving you, here is a comparison of a lunchbox made entirely of individually packaged foods versus one made from larger portions divided into the same-sized individual portions.

Individually wrapped	Cost of larger size divided into same sized portions*
2 individually wrapped cheeses	58% less
Chopped melon	64% less
Packet of root vegetable crisps	6% less
Fruit yogurt pouch	40% less
Packet of olives	78% less

*calculated using Ocado online store, using comparable products March 2019.

Not only does it make sense to buy larger portions then decant the food into smaller containers, it also makes sense in some cases to make your own version at home. Let's look at a few examples:

Make your own versions

Shop-bought popcorn versus made-at-home: Just 1 tablespoon of kernels would yield 3 shop-bought bags.

Kale chips: Shop-bought kale chips can be as much as one hundred times the price of raw kale per 100g of product.

Shop-bought salads: Can be up to three times the cost of the ingredients in the salad.

With a little time and planning at home you can benefit your pocket and the environment by making home-made versions of shop-bought or café/canteen-prepared meals and desserts. Many examples are covered in the chapters of this book and include:

- Yogurt-based desserts and alternatives to yogurt
- Hot meals to take to school or work in a flask (or leftovers to take to school or work – an even better way to reduce food waste and save money)
- Smoothies to take to school or work in an insulated flask
- Alternatives to crisps
- Vegetable- and fruit-based dishes for lunches
- Alternatives to sandwiches
- Soups

The ingredients required to make many dishes that are ideal for packed lunches don't cost anywhere near as much as they would from a shop. Salads, soups, sandwiches, cake slices inevitably cost several times more if you buy them made up and ready to go.

Be in (quality) control

The added benefit of making real-food lunches and packing them thoughtfully is that you are the one who gets to manage quality control, what foods go into the lunch, and ultimately you also get to serve the environment better. Allergies and food intolerances are prevalent in our society and so too are health conditions that improve when certain foods are eliminated. Some simply prefer certain foods or follow a particular way of eating, such as vegetarian or paleo. Making your own lunches means you can be in control of what ingredients do and don't make it into your lunchbox. That way there's also less food wasted as everything gets eaten.

Of course, what makes these lunches even more cost-effective and environmentally friendly is using reusable and durable packaging. Check out the TRANSPORTING LUNCH TO WORK OR SCHOOL chapter (p.21) to find out more.

What to do if your child gets bullied for having a healthy lunch

Others Commenting on Your Child's Lunch

'Other children are mean to my child because his lunch is healthy.'

'Some children call my child's food horrible names because they've never seen or heard of it before!'

'The children at my daughters' school don't like the reusable packaging we use.'

These are a few of the statements I have heard and been asked about over the years. While it is a shame that eating healthier food and being more adventurous than the standard white bread ham sandwich, crisps and a chocolate bar is seen as odd or strange, it is something that other children may comment on simply because they're uncertain how to react to something different from the perceived norm.

It is often the case in life that people fear what they do not know. For others they are jealous that they don't get packed anything more adventurous than the standard fare. In these cases, your children might feel like unwilling ambassadors for healthier foods, but it is well worth sticking to your guns because it may well help others understand the value of healthier foods for energy, concentration and for boosting the immune system. Often it is only a matter of time before the comments subside, and in fact ultimately many are more intrigued than fearful. In my experience I often find other children, parents and even teachers start to ask about foods and ingredients because they too would like to enjoy some healthier options.

But Branded Items are 'Cool'!

We will all be familiar with the allure of brightly coloured food packaging featuring familiar cartoon characters, or a 'free' gift inside. The most appealing packaging and these compelling offers are often on the sorts of foods our children, particularly younger children, find hard to resist, i.e. sugary yogurts, sweetened snack bars, chocolate bars and flavoured crisps. Not having these sorts of foods packed in their lunches can make some children feel different, odd and excluded.

There's one simple way to turn this on its head and that's to use the packaging to help educate your children. The product will have its health value revealed by the nutrition labelling, and even the ingredients. Showing your child a comparable but healthier and unbranded version of their favoured food can help them to understand how much better for their body the unbranded product will be and how they're being influenced by the packaging. Cost might also be a factor in helping your child understand that, for example, for the price of one branded pack of yogurts they could enjoy two healthier unbranded packs. If this doesn't wash, and I am sure at times it won't, then we may need to think about better ways to pack lunches. They too need to be appealing and alluring.

Better Packaging

Lunchbox packaging can make some children feel as though they are different from others. In the same way that popular characters on brightly coloured food packaging is alluring, so lunches packed in cling film, brown greaseproof paper or foil might be deemed boring and uninspiring. The good news is that lunches can be made to look more inspiring and have greater visual appeal with very little effort. Characters on lunchboxes or the latest lunchbox trend might be costly and too expensive for all to follow. However, there are some really cost effective and genuinely cool ways to take lunch to school that could help those who have others make comments on their healthier food.

- Flasks are a winner for some children because nobody can actually see inside; the same applies to insulated drink bottles. So, if your child wants to take soup or last night's leftovers to school and have a healthy smoothie or fruit-infused water to drink, nobody need know, other than from the brief glimpse other children may catch at lunchtime.
- Bento boxes that show all the food on offer in one compartmentalised lunchbox all under one lid are on-trend and practical. Of course, other children will also see what's in the lunchbox, but the box itself is unusual and if they like the look of that, they could well refrain from commenting on the contents.
- For some, the allure of stainless-steel containers is their durability but they also look modern and fresh. They are

admittedly an investment, but over time that investment will pay off. They seal in smells, making cooked eggs or fish for example less obtrusive, and as they are opaque nobody can see what's inside until lunchtime comes.

- A jar (plastic or even glass for an older child) takes the opposite view, i.e. that what you see is what you get. Layered salads with a dressing to add at lunchtime means the contents can be made to be extremely visually appealing. Once again this is a different approach but one that may catch on and win over peers in due course.

Get the School on Board

Many schools have healthy-eating policies and even healthy-lunchbox policies. Schools can help when a child is getting bullied or comments are being made on their healthier lunch. Simply asking the school to be aware of the situation and positively encourage healthy eating as a community is important not just for your child but for others too.

Education can go a long way towards helping other children understand that healthy eating isn't uncool. Healthier foods are what some of the top performing athletes, footballers and TV stars eat to improve their levels of energy and concentration – and look where it gets them!

Helpful Retorts

Over the years of working as a lunchbox expert I have come across some excellent retorts that may help children ward off some of the negative commentary they receive from other children:

1. We cook healthy food at home, so I bring healthy food to eat at school.
2. I have the foods in my lunch that I need to power me through football/hockey/dance/music practice later on today.
3. I am eating for improved energy, concentration and ultimately the best results I can get.
4. Real food can cost less than processed foods, so I am saving money and improving my health at the same time. A win-win!
5. I prefer the taste of real yogurt/bread/cheese/fruit, etc.
6. I simply feel better when I eat this way.

Five packed-lunch tips for parents of fussy eaters

These steps will not only empower your fussy eater and make him or her more likely to eat whatever they take to school, but it also helps prepare them for a time when they will be able to pack their own nutritionally balanced lunches.

Get Them Involved

A lot of parents complain that their child is coming home with a virtually untouched lunch box each day and that they complain about the foods that have been packed for them. As with picky eating at any meal of the day, if a child hasn't been involved in the preparation of the food, they often have very little interest in it. Mornings are busy and stressful, but your child can get involved in preparation even earlier than the morning preparation stage by helping devise a lunchbox menu plan like the one at the beginning of this book (p.12).This can then influence your weekly food shopping list. You will have a range of foods that your child is happy to eat while giving you reassurance that the lunch they're eating is balanced.

In the mornings when there may already be a lot going on in the kitchen you can get the children involved in some simple tasks that help with lunchbox prep. Let your child pull up a chair, grab the biscuit cutters or a child-friendly knife and chop some fruit or vegetables for themselves in the way they would like to eat them. Allow your child to select a few different snacks to go into their lunchbox – this is particularly effective if your picky eater is more of a grazer. Have them help you put their lunch foods into their bento box, fabric sandwich wraps, fabric snack bags or containers, and remind them of the need for a cold pack and cutlery so that one day they will be able to manage this process themselves.

Even having them in the kitchen as the lunches are prepared can be helpful. That way they feel informed and part of the process. As they get older, children can be gently encouraged to get involved more directly, packing their own lunches as and when it works out timing wise. Some children are ready for this at 8, 9 or 10 years old, but others won't be ready until well into their teens.

Pack Their Favourite Foods Plus One Thing New

If you are the parents of a picky eater, then I advise not packing too many new foods at once. That's not to say new foods cannot be packed at all but just not too many. Children's tastebuds are numerous and susceptible to intense flavours, whereas adults have fewer and so tend not to taste flavours as intensely. This explains why adults are open to a wider variety of tastes and flavours than children. In addition to this, young children don't like change, they prefer routine.

It is worth considering these facts when children start to complain about new foods in their lunches. Packing the mostly familiar with the odd unfamiliar new food is the best strategy. If they like their white bread ham sandwich, fruity yogurt and apple, then suddenly packing a vegetable slice, berry chia pudding and choco-banana milkshake is not going to be well received and all the effort that went into preparing it will be for nothing.

It's also really tempting to try to start over by packing only healthy foods in their lunchboxes, but believe me, this won't work. You must change things little by little over time. Try replacing the yogurt with the chia berry pudding. Vary the berries or fruit used and talk to your child about whether they enjoyed this texture and that flavour. If they like it then perhaps try replacing the sandwich with a vegetable slice a couple of times per week. You can see how this goes. Just don't make packed lunches a battlefield. Moving to healthier, more adventurous lunches doesn't need to be stressful. It's more like a long-term, joint project!

Invest in Suitable Equipment

Bento boxes make it really easy for younger children to open and access all the foods they have packed for their lunch. There are some brands selling bento boxes with words and pictures depicting the different food groups that make up a balanced lunchbox. These really help younger children decide what food to choose from each group, and ensures they are already starting to think in terms of a balanced lunch.

For older children, either a bento box or lots of easy-to-open containers ensures they can see what's been packed and how to get to it.

It is important to allow your child to be involved in choosing the box or containers and then the bag that they take their lunch in. Peer pressure and materialism are rife at school. Be prepared to invest a little in an insulated lunch bag and the box or containers to go with it.

It is an investment but one worth making. If your children are proud and happy with their lunch and the way it is presented, they are far more likely to return empty-handed, with the food having been eaten.

Make Food Easily Accessible

Make it easy for them. Don't make anything too fiddly or pack anything too difficult to eat quickly. Often children want to eat and then get on with the rest of their valuable lunchtime playing outside. My own children have come home with their apples uneaten, and when I ask why they have complained that they took too long to eat! When it comes to fruit and vegetables, you need to make eating them as easy as possible. Time spent chopping fruit and vegetables with your child is time well spent. The food also looks more appealing this way, which is why people are willing to spend so much money on pre-prepared and chopped fruits and vegetables in supermarkets. However, this way of presenting fruit or vegetables is costly both to you and the environment. There are some really simple ways to present vegetables and fruit that make it far more likely for your picky eater to want to eat them:

- Soups served with bread, pasta or noodles that soak up a lot of the liquid allow for it to be eaten more easily.
- Dividing crunchy snacks into small paper bags means they're easily eaten and the packaging can be disposed of (or easily recycled) at lunch- or break-time.
- Reusable food pouches can be used for smoothies, yogurts and purées (fruit or vegetable or both combined).
- Easy-peel satsumas and bananas are useful and portable.
- Apples can be sliced into wedges using a wedger then held together with an elastic band so as not to go brown.
- Vegetable portions are far more likely to be eaten when served with a dip. A selection of chopped, crisp salad vegetables, such as carrots, sugar snaps, baby sweetcorn, cucumber, celery and peppers, are easy to eat with a dip.

Chill, Chill, Chill

Don't beat yourself up if you feel like you cannot get your child to eat a varied and nutritious packed lunch. So long as your children are getting some real, fresh food in their diet and you are doing your best to introduce them to new foods, don't panic. Most children will eventually get hungry and eat. It's hard not to worry when you think of them being hungry during the day, especially if they are picky eaters. But even picky eaters will usually eat something when their stomachs start to growl!

In the meantime, to summarise, use these five top tips:

1. Mix food choices up but don't change too much too soon.
2. Get the children involved in both the planning and creation of their own lunches.
3. Make sure the equipment they have for taking their lunches to school is suitable and allows easy access to foods.
4. Ensure they can eat the packed foods easily.
5. Relax. They may end up developing a greater interest in food and tasting new items you never expected as a result of all of the above. Getting kids to eat their lunch doesn't need to be a struggle.

14 Real Food Lunches for Life

If in selecting this book to read you were hoping for some real lunchtime food inspiration, then undoubtedly you will have found some new ideas for shop-bought and home-made foods or found a new way to tackle a current lunchbox-packing stumbling block. In reading this book from cover to cover you will have been apprised of almost every aspect of real food lunchboxes, from the planning to the buying, from the packing to the transporting, and you will have learnt how to overcome hurdles and objections along the way.

As we look at the world around us, our focus as human beings is undeniably on making better, healthier food choices not only for ourselves but also for our planet. While different diet fads and opinions around food and eating surround us, and daily attention-grabbing headlines provide misleading nutritional guidelines, one message is loud and clear: real food is better for us than processed. Whether it is the bread you choose to make your sandwich on or the snack you choose to fill your lunchbox with, the opportunity to waste less food by taking leftovers for lunch or by using up vegetables in soups, there are plenty of simple tweaks we could all make to improve our lunches and focus more on real-food lunchtimes.

We've learned throughout this book how some of the lunchbox habits we have fallen into are not helping improve our health and wellbeing in the longer term nor our shorter-term energy, mood and concentration levels. By viewing lunchboxes as a significant and important meal, by thinking food not just fuel, we can start to enjoy greater variety in our lunches. We can also hope for better health outcomes and a healthier planet too.

All that is left for me to do is to wish you enjoyable meals at lunchtime. Do not try to change everything at once. New habits are formed over months, not days. Just one change or a couple of tweaks should be enough to start. Allow these to become the norm then change or tweak something else. Happy lunches!

Jenny Tschiesche, The Lunchbox Doctor

www.lunchboxdoctor.com
FB: www.facebook.com/lunchboxdoctor
Instagram: www.instagram.com/lunchboxdoctor
Twitter: www.twitter.com/jennytschiesche

Index